FRCS Part 2
Paper Critique Handbook

Academic Viva Preparation Guide

Spot the Spin · Read the Chart · Say the Right Words

2026 Edition
"Making the Difficult Easy"
J.R. Morgan
AMaC Publishing

FRCS Part 2 Paper Critique Handbook
Academic Viva Preparation Guide · 2026 Edition
First published 2026 by AMaC Publishing.

ISBN 978-1-0667467-9-8 (paperback)
J.R. Morgan is a pen name.

Disclaimer — please read. This handbook is an examination revision aid. It is not a clinical guideline, a treatment protocol, or a substitute for current national guidance, local policy, or independent clinical judgement. Nothing in it should be used to direct the care of a patient.

Trial results are quoted from the primary publications listed in the References; the book uses no in-text citation numbers. Several worked examples use *reconstructed* figures chosen to illustrate a calculation; these are labelled as such on the page and must not be quoted as trial data. Charts whose footnote carries "Illustrative data" or "constructed teaching example" are invented for teaching and do not report any real study. That footnote is printed inside the figure itself, beneath the chart; several also state the method used and the limits of the figure in the same place.

Evidence is current to a cut-off of June 2026. Guidelines and trial evidence change; readers must verify against the latest sources before relying on any statement for examination or practice.

Neither the author nor the publisher accepts liability for any loss or damage arising from reliance on the contents of this book, including examination outcomes.

This publication is not affiliated with, endorsed by, or connected to the Royal Colleges of Surgeons, the Intercollegiate Surgical Curriculum Programme, or any examining body. FRCS is used descriptively to identify the examination for which this book prepares candidates.

A CIP catalogue record for this book is available from the British Library.
AMaC Publishing · Manchester, United Kingdom
amac-medical.com

Table of Contents

How to Use This Handbook....1
Three Ways to Study....1
Introduction....3
How This Book Was Produced....4
SECTION 1: Foundations of Paper Critique....5
1.1 Purpose and Format of the FRCS Part 2 Viva....5
1.2 How to Read a Surgical Paper (The 4-Pass Method)....6
1.3 Understanding Study Designs: Quick Overview....8
1.4 Basic Statistics....9
1.5 Bias and Confounding....11
SECTION 2: Research Study Designs Explained Simply....14
2.1 Why Study Design Matters in the Viva....15
2.2 Observational Studies in Detail....16
2.3 Experimental Studies (RCTs)....17
2.4 Systematic Reviews and Meta-Analyses....19
SECTION 3: Statistics & Interpretation....20
3.1 Key Statistical Concepts....20
3.2 Applied Risk Measures (ARR, RRR, NNT, NNH)....20
3.3 Common Statistical Tests....23
3.4 Interpreting Tables....24
3.5 Interpreting Graphs and Charts....25
ADVANCED CONTENT MODULES....77
MODULE 1: Advanced Clinical Chart Examples....77
Example 1: Grouped Bar Chart — Anastomotic Leak Risk Factors....77
Example 2: Scatter Plot — Oncotype DX Score vs Chemotherapy Benefit....81
Example 3: Pie Chart — Distribution of Colorectal Cancer Presenting Features. 84
Example 4: Box Plot — Post-EVAR Quality of Life Scores....88
Example 5: ROC Curve — Predicting Symptomatic Carotid Stenosis....90
Example 6: Funnel Plot — Publication Bias in Liver Resection Meta-Analysis....94
MODULE 2: Advanced Statistical Concepts....98
Card 1: The Proportional Hazards Assumption....98
Card 2: Non-Inferiority vs Superiority Trials....99
Card 3: ITT vs Per-Protocol Analysis....101
Card 4: Multiple Testing Problem & Corrections....103
Card 5: Confounding vs Effect Modification....105
Card 6: Survival Analysis — Key Concepts....107

Card 7: Publication Bias — Detection & Impact....109
Card 8: Bayesian vs Frequentist Interpretation....111
REFERENCE SECTION A: Study Design Cards....113
Card 9: Adaptive Trial Designs....113
Card 10: Cluster Randomised Trials....114
Card 11: Crossover Trial Designs....116
Card 12: Propensity Score Matching....118
REFERENCE SECTION B: Critical Appraisal Checklists....121
Card 13: CONSORT Checklist (RCTs) — Essential Items....121
Card 14: PRISMA Flowchart (Systematic Reviews)....123
Card 15: Risk of Bias 2.0 Tool (RoB 2)....125
Checkpoint: the foundations are laid....126

SECTION 4: Step-by-Step Paper Critique Framework....127
4.1 The PICO Framework....128
4.2 Your Opening Statement....128
4.3 Methods Assessment Checklist....129
4.4 Results Framework....130
4.5 Critique Structure....131
4.6 Mock Viva Example: MAGIC Trial....132

SECTION 5: Practice Papers — Full Model Critiques....135
5.1 CROSS Trial — Oesophageal Cancer....135
5.2 MAGIC Trial — Gastric Cancer (Summary; full critique in Section 4.6)....138
5.3 ACOSOG Z0011 Trial — Breast Surgery....138
5.4 Dutch TME Trial — Rectal Cancer....141

Interlude — A Messier Paper: The RPI Study....144
The Model Viva Answer....146
Ask Yourself....147

SECTION 6: Viva Checklists & Exam Technique....149
6.1 Complete Viva Checklist....149
6.2 Time Management Strategy....150
6.3 Professional Language — The SBAR Technique....151
6.4 Common Traps and How to Avoid Them....151
6.5 The Examiner's Fork — What the Question Is Primarily Testing....154
6.6 Phrases to Use and Avoid....155
6.7 Body Language and Presentation....156
6.8 Delivering the Answer Under Pressure....157

APPENDIX A: Quick Reference Tables....158
Study Design Comparison at a Glance....158

P-Values and Confidence Intervals Quick Guide.....158
Risk Measures Formula Card.....159

APPENDIX B: Statistical Tests Summary.....160

Choosing the Right Test.....160
Statistical Test Selector — Visual Decision Tree.....161
Understanding Regression Types.....162

APPENDIX C: Bias Types Reference.....163

Comprehensive Bias Table.....163

APPENDIX D: Last 48 Hours Revision Pack.....165

Revision Timeline Grid — Choose Your Strategy.....165
Must-Know Trials by Specialty.....166
Statistical Concepts — Memory Joggers.....167
Final Checklist — Night Before Exam.....168
Emergency Phrases if You're Struggling.....168

APPENDIX E: The Glossary of Spin.....169

1 · When the primary outcome failed.....169
2 · When the statistics are being nudged.....170
3 · When generalisability is being oversold.....170
4 · When safety and durability are being stretched.....171
5 · When the framing is doing the persuading.....171

APPENDIX F: Test Yourself.....173

Exercise 1.....173
Exercise 2.....173
Exercise 3.....174
Exercise 4.....175
Exercise 5.....175
Exercise 6.....176
Exercise 7.....176
Exercise 8.....177

Index.....178

Quick Reference Card — Exam Day!.....181

References.....183

About the Author.....187
About This Book.....187
Good Luck!.....187

List of Charts

Chart A. Kaplan–Meier Survival Curves....26
Chart B. Forest Plots (Meta-Analysis)....29
Chart C. Bar Charts — Comparing Groups....32
Chart D. 2×2 Contingency Tables....36
Chart E. Pie Charts — Distribution Analysis....38
Chart E2. Stage at Diagnosis — Ordered Categories....42
Chart E3. Mode of Presentation — Screening and Survival Bias (within Example 3)....85
Chart F. Box Plots (Box-and-Whisker Plots)....43
Chart G. Scatter Plots with Regression Line....47
Chart H. ROC Curves — Diagnostic Test Performance....52
Chart I. Funnel Plots — Publication Bias in Meta-Analysis....56
Chart J. CONSORT Flow Diagram — Where Patients Are Lost....61
Chart K. PRISMA Flow Diagram — How a Review Was Assembled....63
Chart L. Cumulative Incidence — Competing Risks....65
Chart M. Calibration Plot — Do Predicted Risks Match Reality?....67
Chart N. Subgroup Forest Plot — The Commonest TRAP....69
Chart O. Institutional Funnel Plot — Outcome Monitoring....71
Chart P. Bland–Altman Plots — Agreement, Not Correlation....73

List of Cards

Card 1: The Proportional Hazards Assumption....98
Card 2: Non-Inferiority vs Superiority Trials....99
Card 3: ITT vs Per-Protocol Analysis....101
Card 4: Multiple Testing Problem & Corrections....103
Card 5: Confounding vs Effect Modification....105
Card 6: Survival Analysis — Key Concepts....107
Card 7: Publication Bias — Detection & Impact....109
Card 8: Bayesian vs Frequentist Interpretation....111
Card 9: Adaptive Trial Designs....113
Card 10: Cluster Randomised Trials....114
Card 11: Crossover Trial Designs....116
Card 12: Propensity Score Matching....118
Card 13: CONSORT Checklist (RCTs) — Essential Items (CONSORT 2010 items; the 2025 update revises several — check which version a paper reports against)....121
Card 14: PRISMA Flowchart (Systematic Reviews)....123
Card 15: Risk of Bias 2.0 Tool (RoB 2)....125

List of Worked Examples

UPPER GI SURGERY

Example 1: Grouped Bar Chart — Anastomotic Leak Risk Factors....................77

BREAST SURGERY

Example 2: Scatter Plot — Oncotype DX Score vs Chemotherapy Benefit........81

COLORECTAL SURGERY

Example 3: Pie Chart — Distribution of Colorectal Cancer Presenting Features 84

VASCULAR SURGERY

Example 4: Box Plot — Post-EVAR Quality of Life Scores.....................................88

Example 5: ROC Curve — Predicting Symptomatic Carotid Stenosis................90

HPB SURGERY

Example 6: Funnel Plot — Publication Bias in Liver Resection Meta-Analysis 94

How to Use This Handbook

Three Ways to Study

Method 1: Complete Study Programme (6-8 Weeks)

For candidates starting early with time for comprehensive preparation:

1. Week 1-2: Read Section 1 (Foundations) thoroughly. Master the 4-pass reading method and basic statistics.
2. Week 3-4: Study Section 2 (Study Designs) and Section 3 (Statistics), including the risk measures. Practise with the examples provided.
3. Week 5-6: Work through Section 4 (Framework) and all Practice Papers in Section 5. Do full mock vivas.
4. Last week: Master Section 6 (Exam Technique). Practise with colleagues using the checklists.
5. Final 48 hours: Use Appendix D (Last 48 Hours Pack) for final revision.

Method 2: Rapid Preparation (2-3 Weeks)

For candidates closer to exam date who need focused preparation:

1. Days 1-3: Speed-read Section 1, focus on 3.2 (Risk Measures) and 3.5 (Interpreting Graphs)
2. Days 4-7: Master the Step-by-Step Framework (Section 4)
3. Days 8-14: Work through all Practice Papers (Section 5) — one per day
4. Days 15-21: Memorise Viva Checklists (Section 6) and practise with Appendix A-B
5. Final 48 hours: Use Appendix D exclusively

Method 3: Emergency Revision (Last 48 Hours)

For last-minute revision or confidence boosting:

1. Go directly to **Appendix D: Last 48 Hours Revision Pack**
2. Memorise the Quick Reference Tables in **Appendix A**
3. Review the Complete Viva Checklist in **Section 6.1**
4. Read through one Practice Paper that matches your specialty

> **TOP TIP**
> Whatever your timeline, prioritise these three elements:
> 1. The Step-by-Step Framework (Section 4) — this gives you structure
> 2. Risk measures (ARR, RRR, NNT) — these come up in every viva
> 3. One complete Practice Paper from your specialty — for confidence

FRAMEWORK, NOT SCRIPT — read this before the model answers and adapt them, don't recite them

This handbook gives you fully-worked, word-for-word viva answers. They are **scaffolding, not a script.** Their job is to show you the *shape* of a strong answer — the order, the emphasis, the phrases that land — so that the structure becomes second nature.

But examiners have heard the polished, rehearsed answer many times, and a candidate who recites verbatim can sound like they are performing rather than thinking. The deeper risk is not sounding rehearsed but being brittle: a memorised answer breaks the moment the examiner varies the question. Learn the answer to "what is the most important limitation here" and you may have nothing ready when you are asked for the most important strength. The trainee who scores highest is the one who has internalised the method and then speaks in their own words, about the paper actually in front of them. One practical rule for the lists in this book: under pressure, choose the three highest-yield points and develop them properly rather than reciting all eight. An examiner rewards the candidate who explains why a limitation matters, not the one who inventories every limitation. So use the model answers to learn the moves — then close the book and practise saying it your way, out loud, until the structure survives without the words. The Test Yourself set (Appendix F) is built for exactly this.

Introduction

Evidence currency: This 2026 Edition reflects evidence and Intercollegiate examination standards current to mid-2026. The ESOPEC trial (Hoeppner, NEJM 2025) is incorporated into the CROSS critique, and the current JCIE 4–8 marking scheme is used throughout. Evidence cut-off: June 2026.

The FRCS Part 2 Academic Viva can feel overwhelming. You are given 30 minutes with a complex surgical paper, then 15 minutes of questioning by examiners who seem to know every statistical test ever invented.

But here's the secret: **they're not testing your statistics degree**. They're testing whether you can be a safe, critical surgeon who can evaluate research and apply it to patient care.

Who this handbook is for. This book is written for the UK Intercollegiate FRCS (JCIE) Section 2 academic viva, and its worked examples are drawn from the *General Surgery* curriculum — upper GI, colorectal, breast, vascular and HPB. The appraisal method is deliberately transferable: the framework, the statistics, the spin detection and the viva language apply to any specialty FRCS. The examination format does not. Preparation time, oral length and the source material all vary between specialties — Vascular Surgery, for example, sets its Academic Foundation from a published list of landmark trials determined by the SAC rather than from an unseen paper, so there is no reading period at all (JCIE Policy SR13 v8.0, Aug 2025). If you are sitting a specialty other than General Surgery, take the framework and the statistics from this book but confirm the current format for your own examination against JCIE guidance.

What This Handbook Does Differently

Most resources throw statistics textbooks at you. We take a different approach:

1. **Structure over Memory:** We give you frameworks, not facts to memorise
2. **Viva-Ready Language:** Every concept comes with exact phrases to use in the exam
3. **Real Papers, Real Questions:** We use actual landmark trials and show you how examiners question them
4. **Progressive Complexity:** Start simple, build confidence, then tackle the harder stuff

> **WHAT EXAMINERS REWARD**
>
> Defining 'heterogeneity' perfectly is not what earns the mark. What does: spotting when a trial's results do not apply to your patients, and explaining why a p-value of 0.048 might not actually matter.

How Papers Are Selected for Your Viva

Papers set for the academic viva are typically:

- Published in major journals (Lancet, NEJM, BMJ, BJS, Ann Surg)
- Relevant to general surgery or your chosen specialty
- Recent enough to be topical (usually within 5-10 years)
- Contain learning points about study design or methodology
- Have clear clinical applications

This handbook prepares you for all these scenarios.

How This Book Was Produced

This handbook was written by the author. Large language models were used as an editorial and development aid to help refine, improve, structure and critically review aspects of the manuscript.

The author retained responsibility for the content, clinical interpretation, statistical interpretation, examination strategy and all final editorial decisions.

Trial data and references have been checked against the primary publications cited. Worked examples using reconstructed figures are labelled as such on the page and should not be quoted as trial data.

Final responsibility for the accuracy and appropriateness of the content rests with the author.

— AMaC Publishing

SECTION 1: Foundations of Paper Critique

1.1 Purpose and Format of the FRCS Part 2 Viva

What the Examiners Are Looking For

The Academic Viva tests three core competencies:

1. **Critical Appraisal Skills** — Can you identify strengths and weaknesses in research methodology?
2. **Statistical Understanding** — Can you interpret results and determine clinical significance?
3. **Clinical Application** — Can you apply research findings to patient care?

VIVA FORMAT

Reading Time: 30 minutes with the paper (one generic paper relevant to the wider field of General Surgery)

Examination Time: 15 minutes, forming one half of a 30-minute Oral 4 (paired with Special Interest Basic Principles)

Marking (current Intercollegiate 4–8 scale):

Score (Basic Knowledge domain)	Descriptor
8	Excellent basic knowledge; knows the breadth and depth of the topic; provided supporting evidence to a high level
7	Good basic knowledge; comfortable with difficult problems; provided some supporting evidence
6	**Competent knowledge; no major errors; safe practice**
5	Gaps in knowledge; demonstrated a lack of understanding; failed in major competences
4	Poor knowledge; lack of understanding to a level of concern; failed in most or all competences

The descriptors above are those for the Basic Knowledge domain; each of the four domains is rated separately on the same scale. On the JCIE 4–8 scale, a score of **6** is defined as *"competent knowledge, no major errors, safe practice"* — the level a passing candidate is expected to demonstrate. The published JCIE standard is that candidates *"will be examined to the level of a Day 1 Consultant (ST8) in their declared Special Interest"* (JCIE Policy SR5 v8.0, Aug 2025). Performance is judged across the four domains (Basic Knowledge,

Higher Order Processing, Clinical Skills, Professionalism). In practice the pass standard corresponds to consistently reaching 6, but the global judgement is holistic rather than a simple average: a weak domain can still pull an otherwise strong performance to a borderline outcome.
Note: the "4–8, pass mark 6" shorthand is widely used, but the JCIE marking descriptors give separate descriptors for each of the four domains and state the *descriptors* for each score and the "day-one consultant" standard rather than publishing an explicit numeric pass threshold per domain. Examination regulations are also revised periodically. Candidates should confirm the current marking scheme and standard-setting against the latest Intercollegiate (JCIE) guidance for their sitting.

Typical Question Progression

The viva typically follows this pattern:

1. **Opening (2 min):** "Tell me about this paper" — broad overview
2. **Study Design (3 min):** Questions about methodology, randomisation, blinding
3. **Results (4 min):** Interpreting tables, graphs, p-values, confidence intervals
4. **Critique (3 min):** Strengths, limitations, bias
5. **Application (3 min):** How would this change your practice?

1.2 How to Read a Surgical Paper (The 4-Pass Method)

You are given 30 minutes with the paper — far more than most candidates expect, and more than enough to prepare properly rather than merely read. The temptation is to read slowly three times over. Resist it. Use the time in four deliberate passes, the last of which is the one that wins marks:

Pass 1: Orientation (0–4 minutes)

WHAT TO LOOK FOR:

- **Title & Abstract:** What's the research question? What's the answer?
- **Study Design:** Is it RCT, cohort, case-control, systematic review?
- **Numbers:** How many patients? What are the main results?
- **Conclusion:** What do the authors claim?

Pass 2: Interrogation (4–16 minutes)

Focus on these key areas:

IN METHODS:

- Inclusion/exclusion criteria — who was included and why?

- Randomisation method — was it adequate?
- Blinding — who was blinded (patient, surgeon, assessor)?
- Primary outcome — what's the main thing they measured?
- Sample size calculation — did they plan adequately?

IN RESULTS:

- Patient flow diagram — how many dropped out and why?
- Baseline characteristics table — were groups comparable?
- Main results table — what are the p-values and confidence intervals?
- Any subgroup analyses — treat these with suspicion

Pass 3: Construction (16–24 minutes)

This is no longer note-taking — you are drafting what you will actually say. Write the answers out:

1. What are 2-3 **strengths** of this study?
2. What are 2-3 **limitations** or sources of bias?
3. Do the results apply to **my patients**?
4. What would I tell a patient about these findings?

> **Viva Phrases You Can Use:**
> "This is a [study type] published in [journal] in [year], investigating [research question] in [population]."
> "The key finding was [main result], with a p-value of [X] and confidence interval of [Y]."
> "The main strength is [X], but a significant limitation is [Y], which affects the generalisability to [our population]."

Pass 4: Rehearsal (24–29 minutes)

This pass does not exist in most candidates' preparation, and it is the single biggest advantage the 30-minute period gives you. You have already worked out what you think. Now practise saying it.

- **Say the opening summary silently, end to end.** If it does not come out fluently in your head, it will not come out fluently aloud. Fix the sentence now, not in the room.
- **Anticipate the first two questions.** After your summary, the examiner will most often probe the primary outcome or the biggest weakness. Have the first sentence of each answer ready.
- **Choose the one number you will quote.** A single figure delivered precisely — an NNT, a hazard ratio with its confidence interval — does more than five recited approximately.
- **Decide how you want to finish.** Know the sentence you will end on if asked whether you would change your practice. That is usually the last thing an examiner hears before marking.

Leave the final minute unused. It is contingency — for the paragraph you misread, the table you want to check once more, or simply to arrive composed rather than still writing.

1.3 Understanding Study Designs: Quick Overview

Levels of evidence — the Oxford CEBM 2009 framework (and a word on GRADE)

Level	Study type
1a	Systematic review of RCTs
1b	Individual RCT with a narrow confidence interval (the 2011 revision dropped the a/b letter suffixes; they are retained here because examiners still use them)
1c	"All-or-none" (an effect so large no trial is needed — rare in surgery)
2a–2b	Systematic review of cohort studies / an individual cohort study
3	Case-control studies
4	Case series
5	Expert opinion or mechanism-based reasoning

Viva phrase: "This is Level 1b evidence — an individual RCT; a systematic review of such trials would be Level 1a." Note that 1a/1b belongs to the pre-2011 Oxford scheme; the 2011 revision dropped the letter suffixes. Better still, say why the evidence is strong or weak — design, blinding, allocation concealment, follow-up, applicability — rather than reaching for a label.

On GRADE: some examiners reference GRADE instead, which rates the *certainty* of evidence (high / moderate / low / very low) and keeps that separate from the *strength* of recommendation. Whichever label the examiner uses, frame your answer around the same core appraisal — design, bias, magnitude, and applicability — and you will be answering both.

Research studies fall into two broad categories:

1. Observational Studies (No Intervention)

- **Cohort studies:** Follow groups forward in time (e.g., smokers vs non-smokers → lung cancer)
- **Case-control studies:** Look backward from outcome (e.g., lung cancer patients vs controls → smoking history)
- **Cross-sectional:** Snapshot at one time point (prevalence studies)

2. Experimental Studies (Intervention)

- **Randomised Controlled Trials (RCTs): generally regarded as the strongest design for evaluating treatments, because random allocation balances measured and unmeasured confounders — though a poorly conducted RCT is not automatically strong evidence**
- Quasi-experimental: Intervention without randomisation

QUICK MEMORY AID

Cohort = Forward (Cause → Effect)
Case-Control = Backward (Effect → Cause)
RCT = Randomised intervention

*For detailed study design features, strengths, weaknesses, and when each is appropriate, see **Section 2: Research Study Designs Explained***

1.4 Basic Statistics

P-Values: What They Really Mean

The p-value is the probability of seeing results at least as extreme as observed, assuming the null hypothesis is true.

WHAT TO SAY IN THE VIVA

A p-value of 0.03 means there's a 3% probability we'd see a difference this large or larger if there was truly no difference between the treatments. Note the precise meaning: it is the probability of the data given the null hypothesis — **not** the probability that the result is due to chance, nor the probability that the treatment works. A sharp examiner may probe exactly this distinction.

COMMON MISCONCEPTIONS:

- ~~✗ "p=0.05 means there's a 5% chance the null hypothesis is true" (WRONG)~~
- ~~✗ "p<0.05 means the result is clinically important" (WRONG)~~
- ✓ "p<0.05 means we can reject the null hypothesis at the 5% significance level" (CORRECT)

P-Value	Interpretation	What to Say
$p < 0.001$	Very strong evidence	"Highly statistically significant"
0.001 – 0.01	Strong evidence	"Statistically significant"
0.01 – 0.05	Moderate evidence	"Statistically significant at the 5% level"

P-Value	Interpretation	What to Say
0.05 - 0.10	Weak evidence	"Approaching significance"* or "borderline"
p > 0.10	Insufficient evidence against null	"Not statistically significant"

***"Approaching significance" — handle with care.** A p-value of 0.049 and one of 0.051 carry almost identical evidential weight; 0.05 is a convention, not a biological cliff. A p-value between 0.05 and 0.10 can honestly be described as borderline. It becomes spin the moment it is used to imply the result was positive, or is attached to a *failed primary outcome* to soften the verdict. Describe the p-value; never let "a trend towards significance" stand in for "significant." The same care applies to "highly significant": it describes a small p-value, not a large or important effect. See **Appendix E — Glossary of Spin** for how this exact phrase is misused.

Confidence Intervals (CI): More Informative Than P-Values

A 95% CI means: if we repeated this study many times using the same method, about 95 of every 100 confidence intervals constructed this way would contain the true value. In practice, read the CI as the range of values reasonably compatible with the data — not as a 95% probability that the true value sits inside this particular interval.

HOW TO INTERPRET CONFIDENCE INTERVALS:

For Differences (e.g., comparing two means):

- If CI crosses 0 → not statistically significant at the 5% level; the data remain compatible with no difference, and with a range of other values
- If CI doesn't cross 0 → significant difference

FOR RATIOS (OR, RR, HR):

- If CI crosses 1 → not statistically significant at the 5% level; the data remain compatible with no effect, and with a range of other values
- If CI doesn't cross 1 → significant difference

WIDTH OF CI:

- Narrow CI → precise estimate (large sample)
- Wide CI → imprecise estimate (small sample)

EXAMPLE:

Hazard Ratio = 0.68 (95% CI: 0.54-0.86) (illustrative figures)
This means:

- Point estimate: 32% reduction in hazard

- **Viva phrasing:** "The plausible range for the true hazard reduction is 14% to 46%" — this is the correct interpretation. In vivas, "we are 95% confident the true reduction lies between 14% and 46%" is accepted clinical shorthand, though strictly it means: if repeated many times, 95% of such intervals would contain the true value.
- Since the CI does not cross 1.0 (the no-effect line for ratios), the result is statistically significant — the treatment reduces the hazard
- Clinical interpretation: HR 0.68 with CI entirely below 1.0 suggests a meaningful reduction in the rate of the event; combine with ARR and NNT for full clinical picture.
- The intervention appears beneficial

Statistical vs Clinical Significance

> **⚠ CRITICAL CONCEPT**
> **Statistical significance ≠ Clinical importance**
> A huge study might find a "statistically significant" 2% reduction in wound infection rate (p=0.001), but does a 2% absolute difference matter clinically? Probably not.
> Conversely, a small study might show a 20% mortality reduction (clinically massive!) but with p=0.08 because of inadequate power.

> **PERFECT VIVA RESPONSE:**
> "While this result is statistically significant with p=0.002, the absolute difference is only 1.5%, which may not be clinically meaningful. I would need to consider the costs, risks, and patient preferences before changing practice based on this finding."

1.5 Bias and Confounding

Selection Bias

Occurs when the study sample doesn't represent the target population.

EXAMPLES:

- **Volunteer bias:** Patients who agree to join trials may be healthier/more motivated
- **Survival bias:** Only including patients who survived to enrolment excludes early deaths
- **Exclusion criteria too strict:** Trial only enrolling fit patients but results applied to frail elderly

  How to Describe It:
  "There may be selection bias because eligibility was restricted to patients fit enough for the trial intervention, so the enrolled population was

systematically fitter than the patients we operate on. Note that this selection usually operates through performance status or organ function rather than through an age cut-off. This affects the external validity and generalisability of the findings to our population."

Performance Bias

Differences in care between groups other than the intervention being studied.

EXAMPLES:

- Intervention group gets more follow-up visits
- Different surgeons operate on different groups
- One group receives more supportive care

PREVENTION:

Blinding of participants and care providers, standardised protocols for both groups.

Detection Bias

Systematic differences in how outcomes are measured between groups.

EXAMPLES:

- Assessors knowing which treatment was given look harder for complications
- Patients in intervention arm report symptoms more enthusiastically
- Different tests or thresholds used to detect outcomes

PREVENTION:

Blinding of outcome assessors, objective outcome measures, standardised assessment protocols.

Attrition Bias

Systematic differences in withdrawals from the study.

RED FLAGS:

- Different dropout rates between groups
- Missing data not random (e.g., sicker patients drop out)
- Per-protocol analysis instead of intention-to-treat

⚠ EXAM FAVOURITE

If more than about 20% of patients drop out, or if dropout differs appreciably between groups, be ready to discuss attrition bias. Treat those figures as rough warning signs rather than diagnostic thresholds: what matters is how much data are missing, whether the loss is unequal between arms, and above all why patients left. This is a frequent line of questioning.

Confounding

A confounding variable is associated with both the exposure and the outcome, making it appear there's a relationship when there might not be (or masking a true relationship).

CLASSIC EXAMPLE:

Observational study shows coffee drinkers have higher lung cancer rates. Confounded by smoking (smokers drink more coffee AND get lung cancer from smoking, not coffee).

IN SURGERY:

- Comparing open vs laparoscopic surgery, but surgeon experience differs
- Comparing two hospitals, but case-mix differs (one takes sicker patients)
- Comparing two time periods, but management protocols changed

HOW TO CONTROL CONFOUNDING:

Method	How It Works	Example
Randomisation	Randomly allocates to groups, distributing confounders equally	RCTs
Matching	For each case, select control matched on confounders	Match by age, sex, comorbidities
Stratification	Analyse within subgroups of the confounder	Separate analysis for smokers/non-smokers
Multivariable Analysis	Statistical adjustment for multiple confounders	Logistic regression including age, sex, BMI

SECTION 2: Research Study Designs Explained Simply

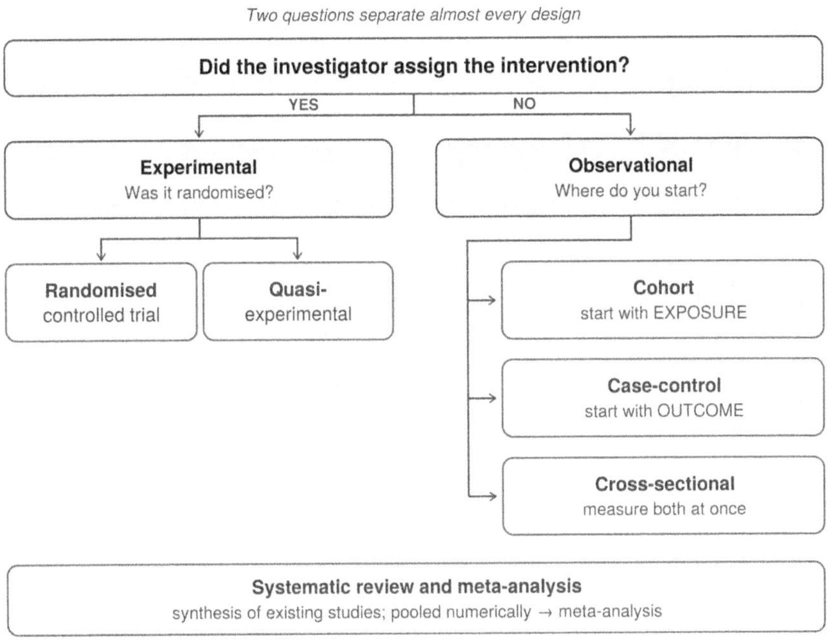

In the viva

- Name the design in your opening sentence — it frames everything after it.
- Cohort studies estimate incidence and can calculate relative risk; case-control studies do not directly estimate incidence and usually report an odds ratio.
- Case-control is efficient for rare outcomes but vulnerable to recall bias.
- A large observational study is still observational; size does not fix confounding.

Colour separates questions from designs. No design here is inferior to another — they answer different questions.

Map 1 · Which study design? Two questions separate almost every design you will meet.

2.1 Why Study Design Matters in the Viva

Study Design Quick Comparison Table

Design	Direction	Key Feature	Best For	Main Limitation	Measure
RCT	Prospective	Random allocation	Testing interventions	Expensive, time-consuming	RR, ARR, NNT
Cohort	Forward (exposure→outcome)	Follow groups over time	Multiple outcomes from one exposure	Cannot control confounding	RR, incidence
Case-Control	Backward (outcome→exposure)	Start with cases vs controls	Rare outcomes	Recall bias, no incidence	Odds Ratio
Cross-Sectional	Snapshot at one time	No follow-up	Prevalence studies	Cannot establish causation	Prevalence
Meta-Analysis	Synthesis of multiple studies	Statistical pooling	Combining evidence	Heterogeneity, publication bias	Pooled estimates

MEMORY AID

Cohort = Forward: "I expose people to X, then follow them to see if Y happens"
Case-Control = Backward: "I find people with Y, then look back to see if they had X"
RCT = Random: "I randomly assign X, then compare outcomes"

The first question after you summarise the paper is almost always: **"What type of study is this?"**

You need to:

1. Correctly identify the design
2. Explain the key features
3. Discuss advantages and limitations of that design

2.2 Observational Studies in Detail

Cohort Studies

DEFINITION

A cohort study follows a group of people over time to see what happens to them. You start with exposure status and look for outcomes.

THE SETUP:

1. Identify exposed and unexposed groups at baseline
2. Follow both groups forward in time
3. Compare incidence of outcomes between groups

EXAMPLE:

Following patients who had laparoscopic cholecystectomy (exposed) vs open cholecystectomy (unexposed) to compare rates of incisional hernia over 5 years.

ADVANTAGES:

- Can calculate true incidence and risk
- Can study multiple outcomes from one exposure
- Temporal relationship clear (exposure before outcome)
- Less prone to recall bias than case-control

DISADVANTAGES:

- Time-consuming and expensive
- Not suitable for rare outcomes
- Subject to loss to follow-up (attrition bias)
- Cannot randomise, so confounding is a problem

> **PERFECT VIVA DESCRIPTION:**
> "This is a prospective cohort study. The investigators identified two groups based on surgical approach and followed them forward over 5 years to compare outcomes. The main advantage is the temporal relationship is clear, but the limitation is we cannot control for confounders like surgeon experience or patient selection. Results are expressed as relative risk."

Case-Control Studies

DEFINITION

A case-control study starts with outcome status (disease/no disease) and looks backward to find exposures. You compare cases (who have the outcome) to controls (who don't).

THE SETUP:

1. Identify cases (people with the outcome)
2. Select controls (people without the outcome)
3. Look back to compare exposures between groups

EXAMPLE:

Patients with anastomotic leak (cases) compared to patients without leak (controls), looking back at risk factors like smoking, obesity, steroid use.

ADVANTAGES:

- Good for rare outcomes (e.g., rare complications)
- Quick and inexpensive
- Can examine multiple risk factors
- Need relatively few participants

DISADVANTAGES:

- Cannot calculate incidence or prevalence
- Prone to recall bias (cases remember exposures better)
- Difficult to establish temporal relationship
- Selection of controls is challenging

> **⚠ COMMON EXAM ERROR**
>
> Don't say "relative risk" for case-control studies! The measure is **Odds Ratio**, not relative risk. Case-control studies cannot directly estimate risk, because sampling is on outcome; cohort studies and randomised trials can estimate risk and therefore relative risk directly.
> Case-control studies and logistic regression report odds ratios (modern papers often report adjusted ORs).

2.3 Experimental Studies (RCTs)

What Makes an RCT an RCT?

Three essential features:

1. **Random allocation** to intervention or control
2. **Concurrent control group** for comparison

3. **Prospective follow-up** to measure outcomes

Types of Randomisation

Method	Description	Advantage
Simple	Coin flip or random number	Truly random
Block	Randomise in blocks to ensure equal numbers	Balanced group sizes
Stratified	Randomise within subgroups	Balance important prognostic factors
Cluster	Randomise groups (e.g., hospitals) not individuals	Practical for intervention at group level

Levels of Blinding

- **Single-blind:** conventionally, the patient does not know the allocation (but the clinician does)
- **Double-blind:** conventionally, patient and treating clinician
- **Triple-blind:** conventionally, patient, treating clinician and outcome assessor

  Use these labels with care: they are applied inconsistently across journals, and "double-blind" in particular can mean any of several combinations. CONSORT recommends stating exactly who was blinded rather than relying on the label. Learn the terms so you recognise them in a paper, but in the viva say who was blinded — patient, operating surgeon, outcome assessor, data analyst — and whether blinding was plausible for that intervention.

IN SURGERY...

True blinding is often impossible (you can't blind a surgeon to whether they did open or laparoscopic surgery!). But you CAN blind:

- The patient (if under GA)
- The outcome assessor (person measuring complications)
- The data analyst

Intention-to-Treat (ITT) Analysis

Analyse patients in the groups they were randomised to, regardless of what actually happened.

EXAMPLE:

100 patients randomised to laparoscopic surgery:

- 15 converted to open
- 5 refused surgery
- 2 died before surgery

- ITT analysis: All 100 analysed in laparoscopic group
- Per-protocol analysis: Only 78 (who completed laparoscopic) analysed

WHY ITT MATTERS

ITT preserves randomisation and reflects real-world practice. If we did per-protocol analysis, we'd only include patients who tolerated the treatment, which gives an overly optimistic result. ITT tells us: 'If I plan to do this operation laparoscopically, what's my overall chance of success?'

2.4 Systematic Reviews and Meta-Analyses

Systematic Review

A comprehensive, reproducible method to identify, evaluate, and synthesise all relevant studies on a topic.

KEY STEPS:

1. Define focused research question (PICO)
2. Comprehensive search of multiple databases
3. Screen studies using predefined criteria
4. Assess quality/bias of included studies
5. Extract and synthesise data

Meta-Analysis

Statistical combination of results from multiple studies to calculate a pooled estimate.

FOREST PLOT INTERPRETATION (SUMMARY)

Forest plots visually display meta-analysis results. Key elements:

- **Each line:** One study (square = estimate, line = CI)
- **Diamond:** Pooled result from all studies
- **Vertical line at 1.0:** Line of no effect
- **I^2 statistic:** Measures heterogeneity (consistency between studies)

VIVA TIP

For detailed forest plot interpretation, heterogeneity thresholds, and model viva responses, see **Chart B in Section 3.5**

SECTION 3: Statistics & Interpretation

3.1 Key Statistical Concepts

Types of Data

Data Type	Description	Examples	Statistical Test
Continuous	Measured on a scale	Age, weight, operative time	t-test, ANOVA
Categorical	Named categories	Gender, ASA grade	Chi-square
Ordinal	Ordered categories	Pain score (mild/moderate/severe)	Mann-Whitney U
Binary	Two categories	Alive/dead, complication yes/no	Chi-square, Fisher's exact

Normal Distribution

Many biological variables follow a bell-shaped curve (normal distribution).

PROPERTIES:

- 68% of data within 1 standard deviation of mean
- 95% within 2 standard deviations
- 99.7% within 3 standard deviations

PARAMETRIC VS NON-PARAMETRIC TESTS:

- **Parametric tests make distributional assumptions — for the t-test and ANOVA, approximate normality within groups, which matters most in small samples**
- **Non-parametric tests avoid that normality assumption but are not assumption-free (Mann-Whitney, Kruskal-Wallis)**

3.2 Applied Risk Measures (ARR, RRR, NNT, NNH)

This section is **GOLD** for the viva. You will almost certainly need to calculate or interpret these.

The 2×2 Table

Most surgical outcomes can be displayed in a simple 2×2 table:

	Outcome Present	Outcome Absent	Total
Treatment	a	b	a + b
Control	c	d	c + d

Key Formulas You MUST Know

1. Event Rate in Each Group

- **Control Event Rate (CER)** = c / (c + d)
- **Experimental Event Rate (EER)** = a / (a + b)

2. Absolute Risk Reduction (ARR)

ARR = CER − EER
The absolute difference in event rates between groups

3. Relative Risk Reduction (RRR)

RRR = (CER − EER) / CER = ARR / CER
The proportional reduction in events

4. Number Needed to Treat (NNT)

NNT = 1 / ARR

> **Critical rule — an NNT is meaningless without its time frame**
> "NNT of 10" says nothing until it becomes "NNT of 10 over five years." Always attach the horizon; examiners are listening for it. Say: "We would need to treat ten patients for five years to prevent one additional event."

How many patients need treatment to prevent one event

5. Number Needed to Harm (NNH)

NNH = 1 / ARI, where the absolute risk increase (ARI) = adverse event rate in treatment − adverse event rate in control

Worked Example: MAGIC Trial

Using MAGIC's real 5-year overall survival (36% with chemo vs 23% with surgery alone), expressed here as the risk of death. *The patient counts in the table below are reconstructed from these survival figures to make the arithmetic concrete — they are* ***not*** *MAGIC's reported death counts, so use them to practise the calculation, not as numbers to quote in the viva.*

	Died	Survived	Total
Chemo + Surgery	160	90	250
Surgery Alone	195	58	253

CALCULATIONS:

CER (Control Event Rate — death in surgery alone):
195 / 253 = 0.771 = 77.1%
EER (Experimental Event Rate — death in chemo + surgery): 160 / 250 = 0.640 = 64.0%
ARR (Absolute Risk Reduction): 77.1% – 64.0% = 13.1% (≈13%)
RRR (Relative Risk Reduction): 13.1% / 77.1% = 0.170 = 17.0%
NNT (Number Needed to Treat): 1 / 0.131 = 7.6, rounded *up* to 8 (round a final NNT up — you cannot treat a fraction of a patient, and rounding up is the conservative direction; this is an approximation based on published 5-year survival rates)

PERFECT VIVA ANSWER:
"The absolute risk reduction is about 13%, meaning chemotherapy prevents death in an additional 13 out of 100 patients at five years. The relative risk reduction is around 17%. The number needed to treat is 8 — meaning we need to treat 8 patients with chemotherapy to prevent one death at five years. While the relative reduction sounds modest, the absolute benefit is clinically meaningful given the poor baseline prognosis in gastric cancer."

Why Both ARR and RRR Matter

⚠ DON'T BE FOOLED BY RRR ALONE!

Scenario 1: Drug reduces mortality from 20% to 10%

- RRR = 50% (sounds amazing!)
- ARR = 10%
- NNT = 10

Scenario 2: Drug reduces mortality from 0.2% to 0.1%

- RRR = 50% (same as above!)
- ARR = 0.1% (much less impressive)
- NNT = 1000

Same RRR, vastly different clinical impact. Always ask for or calculate ARR and NNT!

3.3 Common Statistical Tests

Overview of Statistical Tests

Statistical tests help us determine whether observed differences between groups are likely due to chance or represent real effects. The choice of test depends on:

- **Type of data:** Continuous vs categorical vs survival
- **Number of groups:** 2 groups vs 3+ groups
- **Distribution:** Normal vs non-normal
- **Pairing:** Independent vs paired samples

QUICK RULE
For detailed guidance on which test to use for each scenario, see **Appendix B: Statistical Tests Summary**

Common Exam Error: Correlation is not agreement
Two methods, or two observers, can correlate almost perfectly and still disagree clinically — correlation measures whether values move together, not whether they are the same. If a paper claims two measurements agree, look for a **Bland-Altman plot** for continuous data, or **Cohen's kappa** for categorical judgements such as inter-observer reporting of scans. A Pearson or Spearman coefficient does not answer that question.

Regression Analysis

Regression analysis is used to predict outcomes while controlling for confounders. The type depends on your outcome variable:

- **Linear regression:** Continuous outcomes (e.g., length of stay)
- **Logistic regression:** Binary outcomes (e.g., complication yes/no)
- **Cox regression:** Time-to-event outcomes (e.g., survival)

How do I interpret the regression result?

Linear regression — β. The expected change in the continuous outcome for each one-unit increase in the predictor, with the other variables in the model held constant.

Logistic regression — odds ratio. An OR above 1 means higher odds of the outcome, below 1 lower odds, conditional on the other variables in the model. Remember that an odds ratio is not a risk ratio when the outcome is common.

Cox regression — hazard ratio. An HR below 1 means a lower instantaneous hazard and above 1 a higher one. The hazard ratio should always be read in the context of the proportional hazards assumption: if that assumption does not hold, a single figure summarises an effect that is changing over time (see Chart A and Card 1).

The word that earns the mark: "independent." A regression tells you which factors remain associated with the outcome after adjusting for the others — not which factors cause it, and only for the confounders the authors chose to put in the model.

Key Viva Phrase:
"The authors performed multivariable logistic regression to identify independent predictors of [outcome], adjusting for potential confounders. This allows us to see which factors remain significant after accounting for other variables."

*For detailed regression types and examples, see **Appendix B: Statistical Tests Summary***

3.4 Interpreting Tables

Table 1: Baseline Characteristics

This is always the first table. It shows whether the groups are comparable at baseline.

WHAT TO LOOK FOR:

- **Similar distributions:** Groups should be balanced for age, sex, comorbidities
- **P-values:** Some papers report baseline p-values; CONSORT advises against them, because in a properly randomised trial an imbalance is usually chance. A striking imbalance is still worth noticing — it can point to a problem with the randomisation itself. What matters is whether the imbalanced variable is clinically important and whether the analysis adjusts for it.
- **Sample size:** Are numbers similar between groups?

⚠ RED FLAG
If baseline characteristics differ substantially, this may simply reflect chance (especially in smaller trials), but can also signal a randomisation problem or introduce confounding — the key question is whether the analysis adjusts for the imbalanced variable.

Table 2: Primary and Secondary Outcomes

WHAT TO EXTRACT:

1. **Point estimates** (percentages, means, medians)
2. **Confidence intervals**
3. **P-values**

4. **Effect sizes** (OR, RR, HR)

EXAMINER TIP

I always look at the confidence interval first, not the p-value. If the CI is wide, the result is imprecise regardless of significance. If the point estimate is clinically trivial, I don't care if $p<0.001$.

3.5 Interpreting Graphs and Charts

Visual representations of data are common in surgical papers. You need to interpret them quickly and accurately in the viva. This section provides step-by-step guides for every major chart type.

Chart A. Kaplan–Meier Survival Curves

What you see: A stepped line falling over time, dotted with small "+" tick marks — usually two curves.
What it means: Survival (or event-free) probability over time; each step down is an event, each "+" a censored patient.
Key pattern: Curves that stay apart = a sustained difference. Curves that *cross* are a *visual clue* that proportional hazards may be violated — not proof of it. Confirm formally with the Schoenfeld residuals test ($p<0.05$ counts against proportionality; $p\geq0.05$ is not proof of it) or a log-log plot. If the assumption really is violated, the log-rank test remains valid as a test of whether the curves differ at all, though it loses power when curves cross, because an early benefit and a late harm partly cancel; and a single hazard ratio becomes an inadequate summary of an effect that changes over time.

Viva opener: "This is a Kaplan–Meier curve comparing survival over time; each step is an event and the plus marks are censored patients."

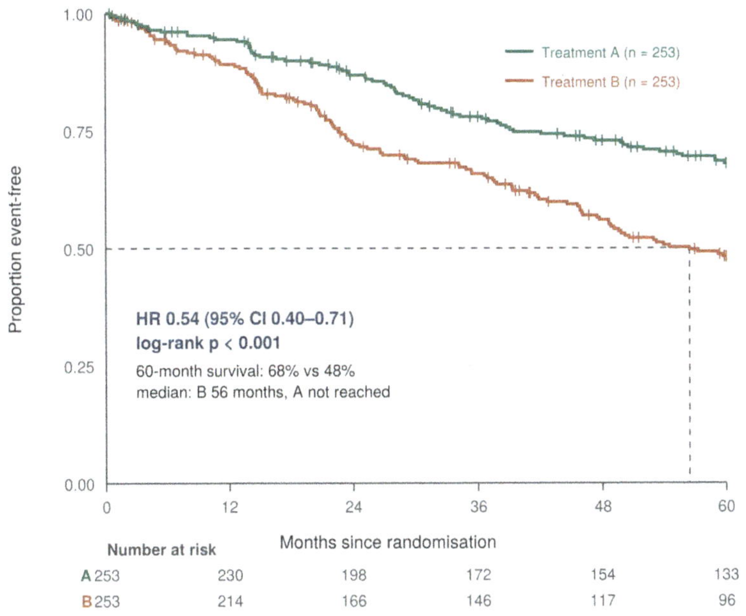

The curves separate early — but who is left at the end?

Illustrative data — tick marks are censored patients. A step's depth depends on how many remain at risk, so a single late death makes a large step. Late estimates rest on few patients and are correspondingly fragile.

Chart A. Kaplan–Meier curves for two treatments, 253 patients per arm. Survival at 60 months is 68% against 48%, hazard ratio 0.54 (95% CI 0.40–0.71), log-rank $p < 0.001$. Median survival is 56 months in arm B and is not reached in arm A. The number-at-risk table shows how thin the data become by 60 months, where 133 of 253 remain in arm A and 96 of 253 in arm B.

Shows the probability of survival (or being event-free) over time.

HOW TO INTERPRET THIS CURVE

1. What Are You Looking At?

A Kaplan–Meier curve shows survival over time.

- The **Y-axis** shows the proportion of patients still alive (or event-free)
- The **X-axis** shows time in months
- Each **"step down"** means a patient died (or had an event)

2. The Step Pattern — Why Steps, Not a Smooth Line?

- Survival only drops when someone dies
- Between deaths, the line stays flat (horizontal)
- This creates the characteristic "step" appearance
- A steeper step or more steps = more deaths = worse survival

3. The "+" Marks — Censored Data

The + symbols (censoring marks) show patients who stopped contributing data before the event occurred. That is not the same as leaving the study: most censoring is administrative, meaning the patient was still event-free when follow-up ended. Others are lost to follow-up or withdraw.

Reasons include: lost to follow-up, still alive at study end, or withdrew consent

These patients contribute data up to that point, then are "censored"

4. Comparing the Two Curves

The upper curve (Treatment A) stays ABOVE the lower curve (Treatment B) throughout follow-up. This means:

- More patients survive in Treatment A at every time point
- The gap between curves represents the treatment benefit
- Where the curves separate matters: early divergence suggests an immediate treatment effect, late divergence a delayed one
- Curves staying separated = sustained benefit

5. The Number at Risk Table — Why It Matters

Look at the numbers below the curve. They show how many patients remain in the study at each time point:

- Both groups start with 253 patients (baseline)

- The numbers at risk decrease over time — pay particular attention to estimates at 48–60 months where remaining patient numbers are small and survival estimates less reliable.
- Fewer patients = less reliable data at later time points
- If numbers drop dramatically, be cautious interpreting late survival differences

6. What to Say in Your Viva

Structure your answer like this:

Step 1 — Describe what you see:
"This Kaplan–Meier curve compares survival between Treatment A and Treatment B over 60 months."

Step 2 — State the key finding:
"Treatment A shows superior survival, with approximately 68% of patients alive at 60 months compared to 48% in Treatment B."

Step 3 — Comment on separation:
"The curves separate early but modestly — about two percentage points by six months — then diverge most sharply between one and two years, reaching a twenty-point gap by five years. The benefit begins quickly and accrues."

Step 4 — Acknowledge limitations:
"The censoring marks indicate patients still event-free when their follow-up ended, whether administratively or through loss to follow-up. I'd want to see confidence intervals and the log-rank test p-value, which is below 0.001."

⚠ RED FLAGS TO MENTION

- **Curves crossing:** If curves cross, treatment benefit may not be consistent over time
- **Wide confidence intervals:** (if shown) indicate uncertainty in the estimate
- **Small numbers at risk:** Late survival estimates based on few patients are unreliable
- **Lots of censoring:** Heavy censoring (many + marks) may introduce bias
- **No p-value shown:** Always ask "Is this difference statistically significant?"

QUICK EXAM-READY SUMMARY

"This Kaplan–Meier analysis demonstrates superior survival in the intervention group (68% at 60 months) versus control group (48% at 60 months). The curves separate early but modestly — about two percentage points by six months — then diverge most sharply between one and two years, reaching a twenty-point gap by five years. Both groups started with 253 patients. The log-rank test gives $p<0.001$, so chance is an unlikely explanation for a separation of this size. I would want to see confidence intervals to assess precision of the estimate."

Chart B. Forest Plots (Meta-Analysis)

What you see: A vertical stack of squares, each on a horizontal line, with a diamond at the bottom and a vertical reference line.
What it means: A meta-analysis: each row is one study (square = estimate, line = CI); the diamond is the pooled result.
Key pattern: Does the diamond cross the line of no effect (1.0 for ratios, 0 for differences)? Then check I^2 for heterogeneity.

> **Viva opener:** "This is a forest plot from a meta-analysis; each line is a study, the diamond is the pooled estimate, and the vertical line is the line of no effect."

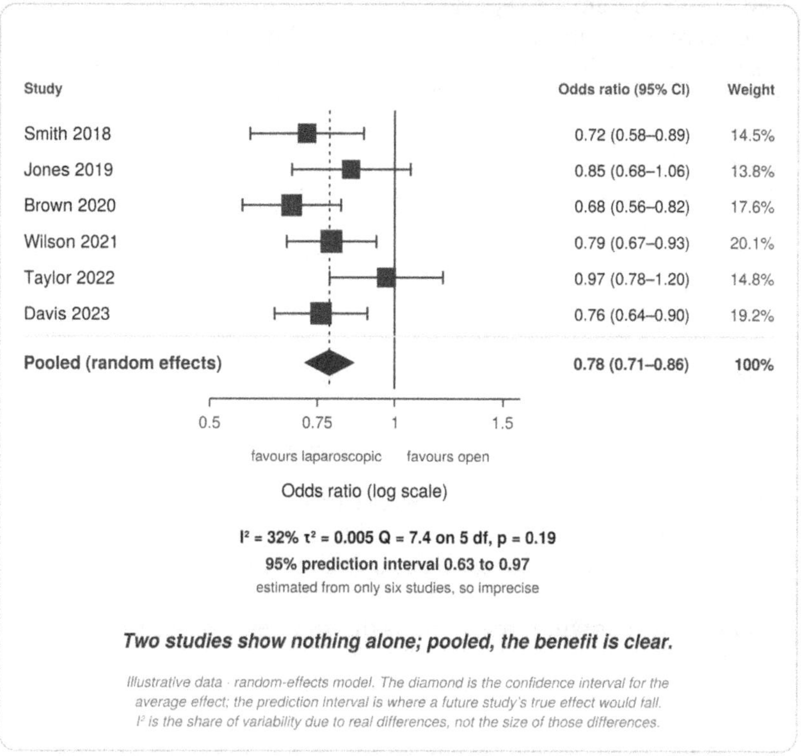

Chart B. Forest plot of six studies comparing laparoscopic with open surgery for mortality. Four studies are individually significant and two are not, yet the pooled random-effects odds ratio is 0.78 (95% CI 0.71–0.86). Heterogeneity is moderate (I^2 = 32%, τ^2 = 0.005). The 95% prediction interval, 0.63 to 0.97, is where the true effect of a future study would be expected to lie.

HOW TO INTERPRET THIS FOREST PLOT

1. What Are You Looking At?

A forest plot visually displays results from multiple studies in a meta-analysis.

- Each **horizontal line** = one study's result
- The **square** = point estimate (odds ratio or risk ratio)
- The **line length** = confidence interval (uncertainty)
- The **square size** = study weight (bigger = more influence)
- The **diamond** at bottom = pooled (combined) result

2. The Vertical Line at 1.0 — "Line of No Effect"

- Left of line (< 1.0): Favours the intervention (laparoscopic)
- Right of line (> 1.0): Favours the control (open)
- Crosses the line: Not statistically significant
- Doesn't cross: Statistically significant

Think of it as: 1.0 = no difference between groups

3. Reading Individual Studies

- Smith 2018: OR = 0.72 [0.58-0.89] — significant benefit for laparoscopic
- Jones 2019: OR = 0.85 [0.68-1.06] — CI crosses 1.0, NOT significant
- Wilson 2021: Largest square (20.1% weight) — most influence on pooled result

Key point: Some studies may not be significant individually, but combined they are!

4. The Diamond — Pooled Estimate (Most Important!)

- The **centre point** of diamond = overall odds ratio (0.78)
- The **width** = 95% confidence interval (0.71-0.86)
- **Doesn't cross 1.0** = statistically significant — for ratio measures (OR, RR, HR); for a mean difference the no-effect line is 0, not 1
- Interpretation: 22% reduction in odds of mortality with laparoscopic surgery

5. Heterogeneity (I^2) — Are Studies Consistent?

I^2 = 32% in this example (moderate heterogeneity). The bands below are rules of thumb, not thresholds — Cochrane describes overlapping

ranges that "may represent" low, moderate or substantial heterogeneity.

- **I^2 < 25%:** Low — studies are consistent, pooling is appropriate
- **I^2 25-50%:** Moderate — some variation between studies
- **I^2 > 50%:** substantial heterogeneity — explore the sources before pooling
- **I^2 > 75%:** very high heterogeneity — pooling needs careful justification and exploration of the causes

Fixed-effect or random-effects? A fixed-effect model assumes every study is estimating one common underlying effect. A random-effects model allows the true effect to vary between studies and estimates an average across that distribution. Where heterogeneity is meaningful, a random-effects model is usually the more defensible choice, and its wider confidence interval reflects that uncertainty rather than concealing it. Do not present it as automatically the better model, though. The choice follows the clinical question — whether you would expect the true effect to differ between these studies — together with the number and character of the studies pooled, not the value of I^2 alone. Two cautions are worth knowing: random-effects models are unstable when there are few studies, because the between-study variance is then poorly estimated; and small studies can receive more relative weight than they would under a fixed-effect model, which matters when small-study effects are present — the problem Chart I is designed to detect.

> **Viva phrase:** "I would not choose between a fixed-effect and a random-effects model from the I^2 value alone. I would ask whether the true effect would be expected to differ across these populations and interventions, and how many studies there are — a random-effects model is unstable when there are few. Here a random-effects model is reasonable, and the prediction interval tells me more than the diamond about what a future trial might find."

6. What to Say in Your Viva

Structure your answer like this:

Step 1 — Describe what you see:

"This forest plot shows a meta-analysis of six studies comparing laparoscopic versus open surgery for mortality."

Step 2 — Comment on individual studies:

"Most individual studies favour laparoscopic surgery, with four showing statistically significant benefit. Two studies (Jones 2019 and Taylor 2022) have confidence intervals crossing 1.0."

Step 3 — State the pooled result:

"The pooled estimate, shown by the diamond at the foot of the plot, is an odds ratio of 0.78 with 95% CI 0.71-0.86. This represents a 22% reduction in odds of mortality with laparoscopic surgery, and the confidence interval doesn't cross 1.0, so the pooled result is statistically significant at the 5% level."

Step 4 — Comment on heterogeneity:
"The I^2 of 32% indicates moderate statistical heterogeneity; pooling appears reasonable here, though clinical and methodological differences between trials should also be considered."
Step 5 — Clinical interpretation:
"This meta-analysis provides high-level evidence that laparoscopic surgery reduces mortality compared to open surgery. Where it pools high-quality RCTs, this corresponds to Oxford Level 1a evidence."

⚠ RED FLAGS TO MENTION

- **High I^2 (>50%):** "The high heterogeneity suggests studies are very different — I'd question whether pooling is appropriate"
- **Funnel plot asymmetry:** May indicate publication bias (negative studies missing)
- **Wide confidence intervals:** Imprecise estimate, need more data
- **Few studies:** with few studies a meta-analysis is less reliable, and tests for funnel-plot asymmetry have low power when studies are few — Cochrane guidance advises against interpreting them below about 10 studies
- **Different populations/interventions:** "Mixing apples and oranges"
- **Diamond crosses line of no effect:** Overall result not significant despite individual significant studies

QUICK EXAM-READY SUMMARY

"This forest plot meta-analysis of six studies demonstrates that laparoscopic surgery reduces mortality with a pooled odds ratio of 0.78 (95% CI 0.71-0.86), representing a 22% reduction in the odds of mortality. The I^2 of 32% indicates moderate heterogeneity, meaning the studies are reasonably consistent. The diamond doesn't cross the line of no effect, so the pooled result is statistically significant at the 5% level. This provides high-level evidence favouring laparoscopic surgery; where a review pools high-quality RCTs, that corresponds to Oxford Level 1a."

Chart C. Bar Charts — Comparing Groups

What you see: Pairs of side-by-side bars repeated across several categories.
What it means: Comparing a rate or value between two groups across categories.
Key pattern: A *consistent direction* across categories is more persuasive than any single bar — and with several categories, watch for multiple comparisons (multiplicity) and missing error bars.

> **Viva opener:** "This is a grouped bar chart comparing two groups across several categories; I'd weigh the consistency of direction and be cautious about multiple comparisons."

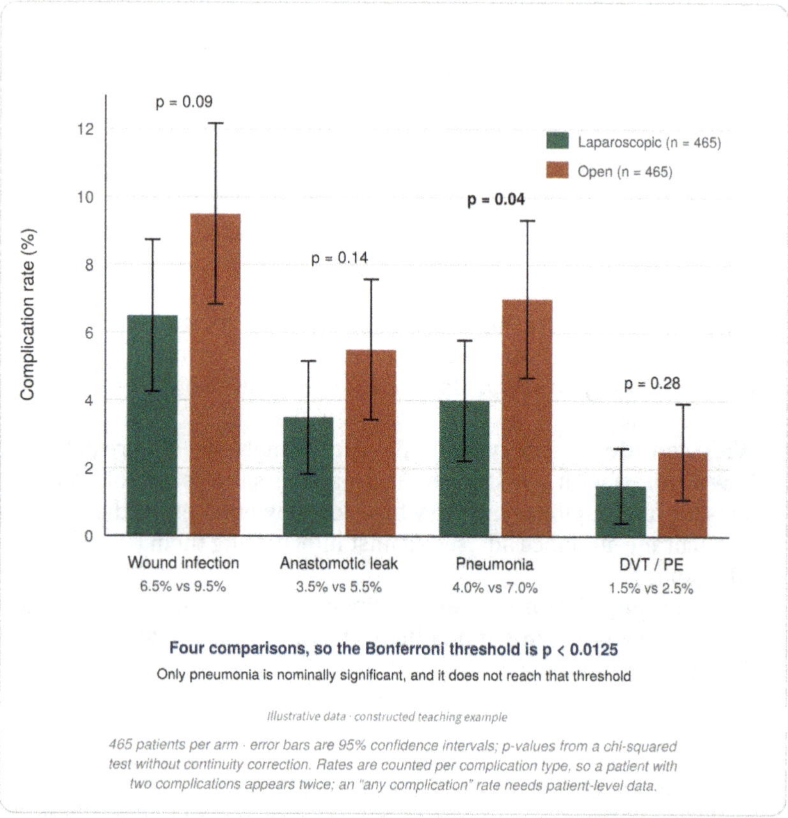

Chart C. Complication rates by type, 465 patients per arm, with 95% confidence intervals. Every category favours laparoscopic surgery, but with 465 per arm only pneumonia reaches $p < 0.05$, and with four comparisons the Bonferroni threshold of 0.0125 is met by none. Rates are exact by construction; with 465 per arm the corresponding patient counts are approximate. The persuasive feature is the consistency of direction rather than any individual p-value — consistent direction, but no single outcome survives correction. Illustrative data · a constructed teaching example, not a real study.

STATISTICAL SUMMARY

Study sample: 930 patients (465 per arm)
Study period: 2020–2023
Complication events: ~186 events across 930 patients (~20% event rate)*
Statistical test: Chi-squared test (per complication type)
Wound infection p-value: 0.09 (not statistically significant)
Interpretation:

Consistent trend favouring laparoscopic across all categories
* Event rate counts each complication type separately; individual patients may have experienced more than one complication. The overall patient rate for any complication is necessarily lower than the event rate, and cannot be derived from this chart — it needs patient-level data. This distinction between event rate and patient rate is itself a viva teaching point — see below.

HOW TO INTERPRET BAR CHARTS

1. What Are You Looking At?

Bar charts compare values across different categories.

- The **Y-axis** shows the measured value (complication rate %)
- The **X-axis** shows the categories being compared (complication types)
- **Bar height** = the value for that category
- **Side-by-side bars** = comparing two groups directly

2. Comparing the Bars — What's Different?

- **Laparoscopic (first bar in each pair):** Lower or similar across all complication types
- **Open (second bar in each pair):** Higher in every category
- **Consistent pattern:** Laparoscopic appears safer across the board
- **Largest absolute differences: wound infection (6.5% vs 9.5%) and pneumonia (4.0% vs 7.0%) — both 3.0 percentage points, so the significant result is not uniquely large — wound infection matches it without reaching significance**

3. Reading the P-Values

- **p=0.09 (Wound Infection): Not significant at the unadjusted 0.05 level**
- **p=0.14 (Anastomotic Leak): Not significant at the unadjusted 0.05 level**
- **p=0.04* (Pneumonia): Nominally significant** at the unadjusted 0.05 level
- **p=0.28 (DVT/PE): No significant difference** — underpowered for this low-event outcome

Key insight — and the trap: Only pneumonia is nominally significant, and four comparisons were made. Correcting for multiplicity (Bonferroni) sets the threshold at p<0.0125 — which even that result does not meet. So the strength of this chart is not a set of independent proofs; it is the *consistent direction of effect across all four outcomes*, which is harder to produce by chance than any single p-value suggests.

4. Clinical vs Statistical Significance

- **Wound infection:** 6.5% vs 9.5% = 3.0% absolute difference (p=0.09) — not statistically significant, but tied for the largest absolute difference and clinically meaningful if real
- **DVT/PE:** 1.5% vs 2.5% = 1.0% absolute difference (p=0.28) — not significant, but in 1,000 patients that is 10 fewer events
- **Viva point:** "DVT/PE doesn't reach significance — likely because the event rate is low and the study may be underpowered for this endpoint. The consistent trend across all four outcomes is nonetheless clinically meaningful"

5. What to Say in Your Viva

Structure your answer like this:

Step 1 — Describe what you see:

"This bar chart compares complication rates between laparoscopic and open surgery across four complication types in 930 patients (465 per arm)."

Step 2 — State the overall pattern:

"Laparoscopic surgery shows consistently lower or similar complication rates across all categories."

Step 3 — Highlight the findings: "Pneumonia is the only outcome reaching nominal significance, 4.0% versus 7.0% (p=0.04). Wound infection (6.5% vs 9.5%, p=0.09) and anastomotic leak (3.5% vs 5.5%, p=0.14) favour laparoscopic surgery without reaching significance, and DVT/PE shows the same direction (1.5% vs 2.5%, p=0.28)."

Step 4 — Clinical interpretation:

"I'd be careful here. Only one of four outcomes is significant at the unadjusted 0.05 level, and with four comparisons a Bonferroni threshold would be p<0.0125, which even that one does not meet. So I wouldn't present these as separate proofs.

What is persuasive is the consistent direction of effect across all four outcomes, which is plausibly a genuine safety benefit — perhaps from gentler tissue handling — but I'd want it confirmed by a pre-specified primary outcome or a larger study before relying on it."

⚠ RED FLAGS TO MENTION

- **Multiple comparisons:** Four tests were run; a Bonferroni correction requires p<0.0125, which even the single nominally significant result does not reach. Treat the individual p-values with caution and lean on the consistent direction instead.
- **Check for error bars: this chart shows 95% confidence intervals, so the precision of each estimate is visible — many published bar charts omit them**

- **Sample size per arm:** Is n=465 adequate to detect differences?
- **Composite outcome missing:** Would be useful to see "any complication" rate

QUICK EXAM-READY SUMMARY

"This bar chart demonstrates consistently lower complication rates with laparoscopic versus open surgery across all four complication types. Pneumonia is reduced from 7.0% to 4.0% (p=0.04), the only outcome reaching nominal significance; wound infection (9.5% to 6.5%, p=0.09) and anastomotic leak (5.5% to 3.5%, p=0.14) point the same way without reaching it. With four comparisons the multiplicity-corrected threshold is p<0.0125, which none meets, so the individual p-values should not be over-read. DVT/PE shows a trend (2.5% vs 1.5%) that does not reach significance (p=0.28), likely reflecting lower event rates. In 465 patients per arm, the genuinely persuasive feature is the consistent direction across all four outcomes, which suggests a real safety benefit worth confirming in a larger, pre-specified study."

Chart D. 2×2 Contingency Tables

What you see: A small two-row, two-column grid of counts (cells a, b, c, d) with row and column totals.
What it means: The raw material for risk measures — event vs no-event, by group.
Key pattern: Event rate in each group first — a/(a+b) and c/(c+d) — then ARR and NNT. Give ARR and NNT, never RRR alone.

Viva opener: "This is a 2×2 table; I'd calculate the event rate in each group, then the absolute risk reduction and the number needed to treat."

The foundation of calculating risk measures — you MUST know how to use these!

EXAMPLE: TREATMENT OUTCOMES IN RCT

	Death	Survived	Total
New Treatment	20 (a)	180 (b)	200
Standard Treatment	40 (c)	160 (d)	200
Total	60	340	400

HOW TO USE 2×2 TABLES

1. Understanding The Layout

- **Rows:** Exposure or treatment groups
- **Columns:** Outcomes (event occurred or not)
- **Cell 'a':** New treatment + Death = 20 patients
- **Cell 'b':** New treatment + Survived = 180 patients
- **Cell 'c':** Standard treatment + Death = 40 patients
- **Cell 'd':** Standard treatment + Survived = 160 patients

> **Memory aid:** "a, b across the top; c, d across the bottom"

2. Calculate Event Rates (CRITICAL STEP)

Experimental Event Rate (EER): EER = a / (a + b) = 20 / 200 = 0.10 = 10%
Control Event Rate (CER): CER = c / (c + d) = 40 / 200 = 0.20 = 20%
Translation: 10% died with new treatment vs 20% with standard treatment

3. Calculate ALL Risk Measures (MEMORISE THESE!)

Absolute Risk Reduction (ARR):
ARR = CER − EER = 20% − 10% = 10%
Meaning: New treatment prevents death in 10 out of 100 patients

Relative Risk Reduction (RRR): RRR = ARR / CER = 10% / 20% = 0.50 = 50%
Meaning: New treatment reduces death risk by half

Number Needed to Treat (NNT): NNT = 1 / ARR = 1 / 0.10 = 10
Meaning: Treat 10 patients to prevent 1 death

Relative Risk (RR): RR = EER / CER = 0.10 / 0.20 = 0.5
Meaning: New treatment patients have half the risk of death

Odds Ratio (OR): OR = (a × d) / (b × c) = (20 × 160) / (180 × 40) = 3200 / 7200 = 0.44
Meaning: The odds of death with the new treatment were 0.44 times those with standard treatment

4. Which Measure to Use When?

Measure	When to Use	Why It Matters
ARR	Always calculate first	Shows actual benefit

Measure	When to Use	Why It Matters
RRR	Comparing effect sizes	Sounds impressive but can mislead
NNT	Clinical decision-making	Most clinically intuitive
RR	RCTs and cohort studies	Can calculate incidence
OR	Case-control studies	When you can't calculate RR

5. What to Say in Your Viva

If shown a 2×2 table and asked to interpret:

Step 1 — Calculate event rates:
"The death rate in the new treatment group is 10% (20 out of 200) compared to 20% in the standard treatment group (40 out of 200)."

Step 2 — Calculate ARR:
"The absolute risk reduction is 10%, meaning the new treatment prevents death in an additional 10 out of every 100 patients treated."

Step 3 — Calculate NNT:
"The number needed to treat is 10, so we need to treat 10 patients with the new therapy to prevent one death over the trial's follow-up period — always state the horizon."

Step 4 — Provide context:
"The relative risk reduction is 50%, which sounds impressive, but the absolute benefit is what matters clinically. An NNT of 10 is very good for a mortality outcome."

⚠ COMMON PITFALLS

- **Don't confuse RR and OR:** the OR approximates the RR when outcomes are uncommon; with common outcomes the OR increasingly overestimates the apparent effect.
- **Don't quote only RRR:** Always give ARR and NNT for context
- **Check the denominator:** Make sure you're using (a+b) and (c+d), not total N
- **NNT for harm:** If treatment increases events, you get NNH (Number Needed to Harm)

QUICK CALCULATION TRICK (APPROXIMATIONS — ROUND UP WHEN QUOTING A FINAL NNT)

If ARR = 10% (0.10), then NNT = 1/0.10 = 10
If ARR = 5% (0.05), then NNT = 1/0.05 = 20
If ARR = 3.3% (0.033), then NNT ≈ 1/0.033 ≈ 30

Memory aid: ARR of 1% = NNT of 100

Chart E. Pie Charts — Distribution Analysis

What you see: A single circle divided into slices.
What it means: Proportions of one whole — parts of 100%.

Key pattern: One dataset only: a pie can't compare two groups (use a bar chart for that). State the sample size, and don't forget the largest slice — often the denominator that puts the rest in perspective.

> **Viva opener:** "This is a pie chart showing the proportions of a single whole; I'd note the sample size and translate the percentages into clinical terms."

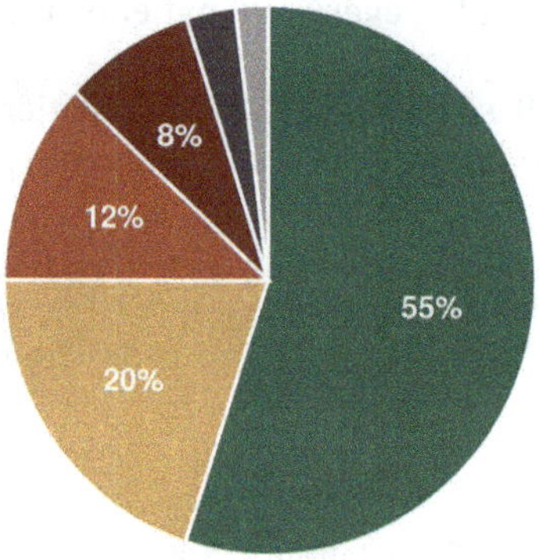

Outcome	%	n
No complications	55%	220
Wound infection	20%	80
Anastomotic leak	12%	48
Pneumonia	8%	32
DVT / PE	3%	12
Other	2%	8
Total	100%	400

Overall complication rate 45% — 180 of 400 patients

n = 400 · each patient is counted once, under their most severe complication, so the slices are mutually exclusive and sum to 100%. Illustrative data: a 12% anastomotic leak rate is higher than most published gastrectomy series.

Chart E. Complications after gastrectomy in 400 patients. A pie chart requires categories that are mutually exclusive, so each patient is counted once under their most severe complication; without that rule the slices would overlap and could not sum to 100%. The counts are given alongside the percentages because a proportion is easier to judge from a number than from an angle.

KEY STATISTICS

Most common: No complications (55%)
Second most common: Wound infection (20%)
Serious complications: 23% combined (leak, pneumonia and DVT/PE)

HOW TO INTERPRET PIE CHARTS

1. What Are You Looking At?

A pie chart shows **PROPORTIONS** — how a total is divided into categories.

- The **WHOLE PIE** = 100% (all 400 patients)
- Each **SLICE** = one category (type of complication or no complication)
- **SIZE** of slice = proportion/percentage
- **LARGER** slice = more common outcome

2. Reading the Slices — What Dominates?

This slice (55%) is LARGEST

- **Good news:** Over half of patients had no complications
- **The second-largest slice (20%):** One in five patients developed wound infection
- **The two mid-sized slices:** anastomotic leak (12%) and pneumonia (8%); with DVT/PE (3%) the serious total is 23%
- **The two smallest slices:** thromboembolic events (3%) and other (2%)

3. Clinical Interpretation

What This Tells You About Gastrectomy Risk

- **Overall complication rate:** 45% (100% - 55% no complications)
- **Most common problem:** Wound infection (20%) — the most frequent, though frequency is not severity
- **Serious complications:** Leak, pneumonia and DVT/PE = 23% combined
- **Life-threatening events:** DVT/PE least frequent in this constructed dataset (3%)

For consent: "There's about a 1 in 2 chance of some complication, though most commonly this is wound infection. More serious problems like anastomotic leak occur in about 1 in 8 patients."

4. What to Say in Your Viva

Structure your answer like this:

Step 1 — Describe what you see:

"This pie chart shows the distribution of complications in 400 patients undergoing gastrectomy."

Step 2 — State the overall pattern:

"The largest slice shows that 55% had no complications, meaning the overall complication rate is 45%."

Step 3 — Highlight key findings:

"The most common complication is wound infection at 20%, followed by anastomotic leak at 12% and pneumonia at 8%. Serious complications —

anastomotic leak, pneumonia and thromboembolism — account for 23% of cases between them."

Step 4 — Clinical significance:

"While the overall complication rate is substantial at 45%, the largest single category is wound infection, which carries different consequences from an anastomotic leak. Serious complications requiring intensive intervention occur in a little under a quarter of patients."

⚠ Red Flags & Limitations of Pie Charts

- **Can only show ONE set of data:** Can't compare two groups (e.g., lap vs open) — use bar chart for that
- **Hard to compare similar slices:** Is 23% really different from 25%? Can't tell precisely
- **Too many categories:** More than 6-7 slices becomes unreadable
- **Missing denominators:** Always state the sample size (n=400)
- **No statistical testing:** Chart doesn't show p-values or confidence intervals
- **Can be misleading:** 3D pie charts distort perception — flat is better

WHEN ARE PIE CHARTS USEFUL IN SURGERY?

- **Complication profiles:** Showing types of complications after a procedure
- **Patient demographics:** Age distribution, ASA grades
- **Tumour stages:** Proportion of patients at each TNM stage
- **Resource allocation:** Where does the budget go?
- **Referral patterns:** Sources of patient referrals

Key principle: Use pie charts when you want to emphasise *proportions of a whole*, not for comparing groups or showing changes over time.

WHAT EXAMINERS REWARD

When presented with a pie chart, candidates often just read the percentages. **The best answers go beyond this** — they translate percentages into clinical language. Instead of saying '12% had anastomotic leak', say 'approximately 1 in 8 patients developed an anastomotic leak, which is a significant concern requiring close surveillance.' This shows clinical reasoning, not just data reading.

Also remember: If the pie chart shows complications, always consider discussing the *no complication* slice — this is the denominator that puts everything in perspective. A 12% leak rate sounds scary, but if — as in this chart — 55% had no complications at all, that's reassuring.

QUICK EXAM-READY SUMMARY

Perfect response for a complication pie chart:

"This pie chart illustrates the distribution of complications in 400 patients after gastrectomy. The largest slice, representing no complications, comprises 55%, giving an overall complication rate of 45%. Wound infection is the most common adverse outcome at 20%, which while important, is generally less severe than anastomotic leak which occurred in 12% or pneumonia in 8%. Serious complications — anastomotic leak, pneumonia and thromboembolism — total 23% between them, so a little under a quarter of patients experienced a major postoperative problem requiring intensive management. This complication profile is consistent with published data for major upper gastrointestinal surgery and would be important information for informed consent."

Chart E2. Stage at Diagnosis — Ordered Categories (n = 500)

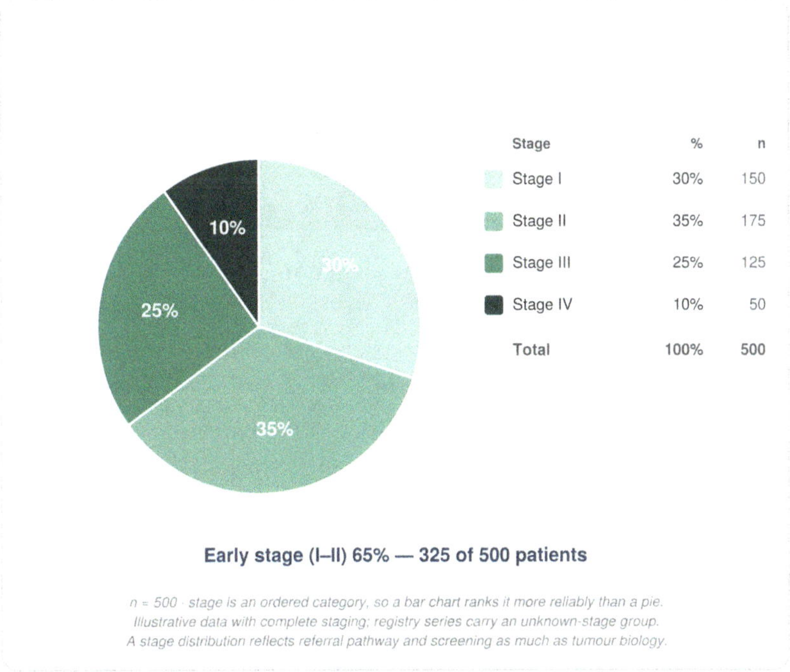

Chart E2. Stage at diagnosis in 500 patients. Sixty-five per cent present with Stage I or II disease, and a further 25% with Stage III, most of whom are treated with curative intent — so the proportion offered curative treatment is considerably higher than the 65% early-stage figure suggests. The shading runs light to dark with advancing stage because stage is an ordered category.

VIVA POINTS:

- **Most common:** Stage II (35%) and Stage I (30%) = 65% potentially curable
- **Advanced disease:** 35% present with Stage III/IV
- **Clinical nuance:** Stage IV (10%, metastatic) is broadly non-curative, but Stage III is frequently resected with curative intent — don't

conflate the two when you read "35% advanced". The curable fraction is higher than that headline implies.

Chart F. Box Plots (Box-and-Whisker Plots)

What you see: A box with a line through it and whiskers extending each side, sometimes with dots beyond.
What it means: The distribution of a continuous variable: median (line), interquartile range (box), range (whiskers), outliers (dots).
Key pattern: The line is the *median*, not the mean; the box is the middle 50%. Compare medians *and* spread between groups.
Viva opener: "This is a box plot showing the distribution of a continuous outcome; the line is the median, the box the interquartile range, and the dots are outliers."

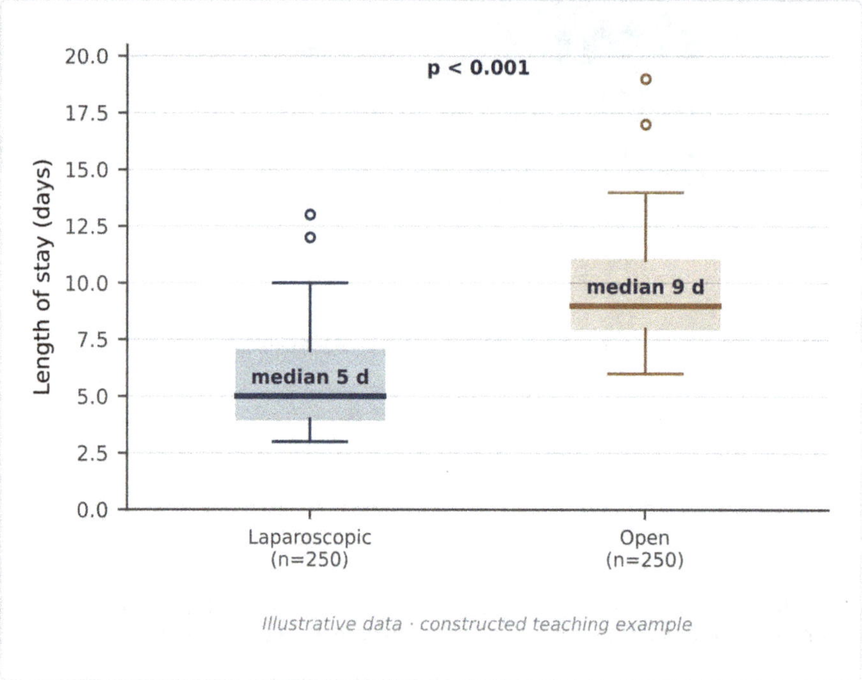

Chart F. Length of stay after laparoscopic and open surgery, 250 patients per arm. The median is 5 days against 9 days, and the boxes span the interquartile range, so half of each group lies inside the shaded band. The whiskers reach the most extreme values within 1.5 times the interquartile range and the circles beyond them are outliers. A box plot shows the shape of a distribution rather than its mean, which is why it suits skewed data such as length of stay.

HOW TO READ BOX PLOTS:

- **Box:** Contains middle 50% of data (interquartile range, IQR)
- **Thick line in box:** Median value
- **Bottom of box:** 25th percentile (Q1)
- **Top of box:** 75th percentile (Q3)
- **Whiskers:** the range of non-outlying values under the plotting convention used — check the legend, since conventions differ (commonly 1.5×IQR, the Tukey convention), though definitions vary between publications
- **Dots beyond whiskers:** Outliers
- **Interpretation:** Laparoscopic shows a shorter median stay with a similar spread

Key Finding: Median hospital stay is 4 days shorter with laparoscopic approach (5 vs 9 days), and the difference in medians is statistically significant ($p<0.001$).

HOW TO INTERPRET BOX PLOTS

1. What Are You Looking At?

A box plot (box-and-whisker plot) shows the **DISTRIBUTION** of continuous data.

- **BOX** = middle 50% of patients (interquartile range, IQR)
- **THICK LINE** inside box = median (50th percentile)
- **WHISKERS** = non-outlying range (commonly 1.5×IQR, the Tukey convention)
- **DOTS** = outliers (unusual values)

Think of it as: A visual summary that tells you the centre (median), spread (IQR), and extremes (whiskers + outliers) all at once.

2. The Five Number Summary

Box plot shows 5 key values (Laparoscopic example):

Value	Position on Plot	Laparoscopic	Open
Lowest non-outlying value	Bottom whisker	3 days	6 days
Q1 (25th percentile)	Bottom of box	4 days	8 days
Median (50th percentile)	Thick line in box	**5 days**	**9 days**
Q3 (75th percentile)	Top of box	7 days	11 days
Highest non-outlying value	Top whisker	10 days	14 days

3. Comparing the Two Groups — What Do You See?

Laparoscopic (left box) vs Open (right box)

A. THE MEDIANS (THICK LINES)

- **Laparoscopic median:** 5 days
- **Open median:** 9 days
- **Difference:** 4 days shorter with laparoscopic (~44% reduction)

B. THE SPREAD (IQR – HEIGHT OF BOX)

- **Laparoscopic IQR:** 4-7 days (range of 3 days)
- **Open IQR:** 8-11 days (range of 3 days)
- **Similar spread,** but open surgery consistently higher

C. THE OUTLIERS (DOTS ABOVE WHISKERS)

- **Laparoscopic:** 2 outliers at 12-13 days
- **Open:** 2 outliers at 17-19 days
- **The most extreme observed values were lower in the laparoscopic group**

4. Statistical Significance – The p-value

p < 0.001 (shown at top)

- This tells you the difference is **highly statistically significant**
- p<0.001 — very strong evidence against the null hypothesis (a difference this large would be very unlikely if the two groups were truly the same)
- There is strong evidence against the null hypothesis of no difference

How they calculated this: Mann-Whitney U test — used to compare two groups when continuous data are non-normal (strictly, it compares whole distributions, commonly interpreted as a difference in medians)

5. What to Say in Your Viva

Perfect structured answer:

Step 1 — Identify the chart:
"This box plot compares hospital length of stay between laparoscopic and open surgery."

Step 2 — State the median values:
"The median hospital stay for laparoscopic surgery is 5 days, indicated by the thick line in the left-hand box, compared to 9 days for open surgery in the right-hand box."

Step 3 — Describe the spread:
"The interquartile range — the height of the box — shows that 50% of laparoscopic patients stayed between 4 and 7 days, whereas 50% of open surgery patients stayed between 8 and 11 days. This demonstrates not only a shorter stay but also consistently shorter across the distribution."

Step 4 — Mention outliers:
"There are outliers in both groups shown as dots beyond the whiskers, representing patients with prolonged stays, which may reflect

complications — though the chart itself cannot establish the cause. The most extreme values were lower in the laparoscopic group."

Step 5 — Statistical significance:

"The difference is highly statistically significant with $p<0.001$, meaning we can be confident this represents a true benefit of laparoscopic surgery rather than chance variation."

Step 6 — Clinical significance:

"A 4-day reduction in median hospital stay is clinically meaningful — it reduces healthcare costs, improves patient satisfaction, and decreases risk of hospital-acquired complications like infections or VTE."

⚠ COMMON MISTAKES TO AVOID

- **DON'T confuse median with mean:** The thick line is the median (50th percentile), NOT the average
- **DON'T ignore the whiskers:** They show the non-outlying range (commonly 1.5×IQR); individual dots beyond the whiskers are outliers
- **DON'T say "all patients":** Say "50% of patients were between..."
- **DON'T call outliers "errors":** They're real patients, often with complications
- **DON'T forget sample size:** Always mention the sample size shown — in this box plot, n=250 per group (500 total)

Why Box Plots Are Better Than Bar Charts for This Data

What a bar chart would hide:

- The distribution shape
- Individual outliers within each group

Box plot shows:

- The median (more robust than mean if there are outliers)
- The spread (IQR)
- The range (whiskers)
- Individual outliers
- Whether data is skewed (if median isn't in centre of box)

Use box plots when: Comparing continuous data between groups and you want to show the full distribution, not just an average.

WHAT EXAMINERS REWARD

Box plots are increasingly common in surgical literature because they convey more information than bar charts. **Strong candidates demonstrate they understand what each part represents.** Don't just say 'the laparoscopic group had shorter stays' — explain using the specific values: 'the median of 5 days versus 9 days, with the interquartile range showing that half of laparoscopic patients were discharged between 4 and 7 days, while half of open surgery patients stayed between 8 and 11 days.'

Also key: If you see outliers, discuss them. 'The presence of outliers at 12-13 days in the laparoscopic group likely represents patients who developed complications. However, even these outliers are shorter than the outliers in the open group, which reach 17-19 days.' This shows nuanced thinking.

⚠ A NOTE ON THE SCRIPTS THAT FOLLOW

These model answers are scaffolds, not lines to memorise. Their value is in the *structure* — the order you move through a paper, the phrases that signal judgement — not the exact words. Recited answers are easy for an examiner to spot, and they collapse the moment the paper in front of you differs from the template. Learn the shape of a good answer, then build your own around whatever you are actually handed. Where an answer offers a list, develop three points well rather than naming all of them.

QUICK EXAM-READY SUMMARY

Perfect 60-second response:

"This box plot compares hospital length of stay between laparoscopic and open surgery patients. The median stay is significantly shorter with laparoscopic surgery at 5 days compared to 9 days for open surgery, indicated by the thick line within each box. The interquartile range — the box itself — shows that the middle 50% of laparoscopic patients stayed between 4 and 7 days, while the middle 50% of open surgery patients stayed between 8 and 11 days. The whiskers extend to show the non-outlying range, with individual dots beyond the whiskers representing outliers — patients with prolonged stays, likely due to complications. This difference is highly statistically significant ($p<0.001$) and clinically meaningful, representing a 4-day reduction in median hospital stay with laparoscopic surgery, with implications for cost, patient satisfaction, and complication risk. The box plot is superior to a bar chart for this data as it displays the full distribution rather than just a mean value."

Chart G. Scatter Plots with Regression Line

What you see: A cloud of dots with a line of best fit through them.
What it means: The relationship between two continuous variables; slope = direction, tightness of clustering = strength (r).
Key pattern: Check *what each dot represents* — a patient, or a group/unit? Group-level dots invite the ecological fallacy. And correlation is not causation. Beware also of Simpson's paradox — a relationship seen in pooled data can reverse once the data are split by an important subgroup.

Viva opener: "This is a scatter plot with a regression line examining the relationship between two continuous variables; I'd confirm what each point represents and remember correlation isn't causation."

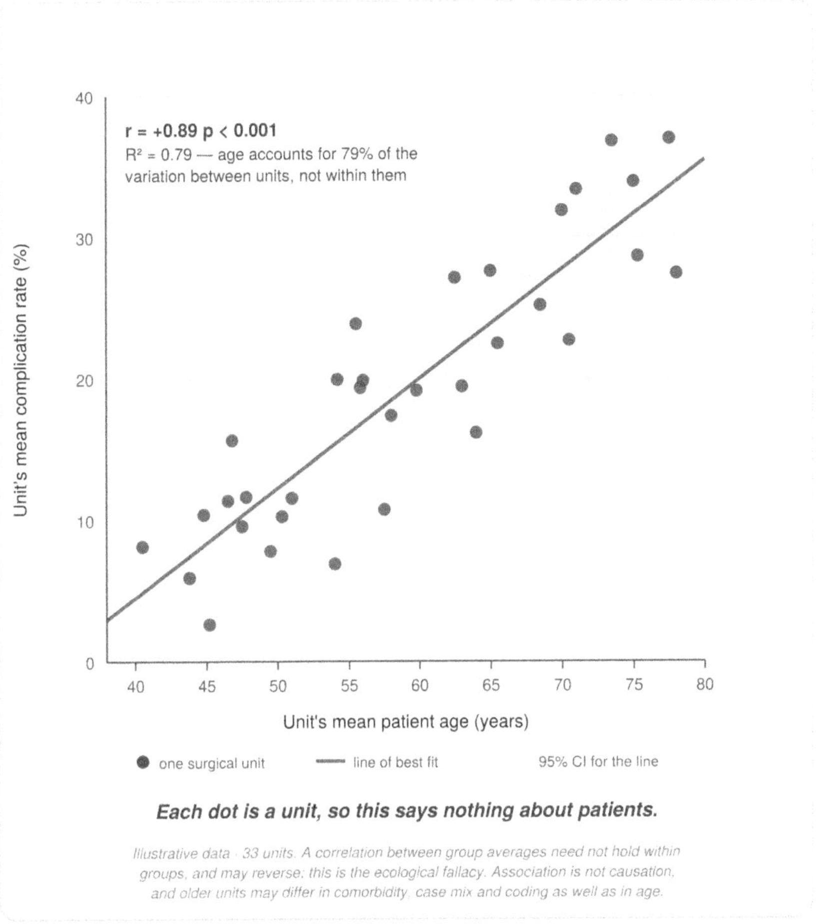

Chart G. Scatter plot with a fitted regression line and its 95% confidence band. Thirty-three units give r = +0.89, so $r^2 = 0.79$: about 79% of the between-unit variation is captured by the fitted line. Because each point is a unit average rather than a patient, the correlation describes units and not the patients within them.

HOW TO INTERPRET SCATTER PLOTS

1. What Are You Looking At?

A scatter plot shows the **RELATIONSHIP** between two continuous variables.

- Each **DOT** = one surgical unit — plotted at that unit's mean patient age and its mean complication rate, *not* an individual patient (there are 33 units here)

- **X-axis** (horizontal) = the unit's mean patient age (predictor variable)
- **Y-axis** (vertical) = the unit's mean complication rate (outcome variable)
- **PATTERN** of dots shows if there's a relationship

2. The PATTERN — What Does It Show?

This shows a POSITIVE CORRELATION

- As age **INCREASES** (moving right) →
- Complication rate **INCREASES** (moving up)
- Dots form an **UPWARD SLOPE** from bottom-left to top-right

Other possible patterns:

- **Negative correlation:** Downward slope (as X ↑, Y ↓)
- **No correlation:** Random scatter, no pattern
- **Non-linear:** Curved pattern

3. The REGRESSION LINE (solid)

LINE OF BEST FIT — the average trend through the data

- Shows the **GENERAL RELATIONSHIP**
- Can be used to **PREDICT** outcomes
- Slope = the rate of change in outcome per unit change in the predictor; strength of association is shown by how tightly the points cluster around the line, not by how steep it is

Reading this line (at the unit level):

- A unit with mean age 40: ~5% mean complication rate
- A unit with mean age 60: ~20% mean complication rate
- A unit with mean age 80: ~35% mean complication rate

Clinical meaning: Roughly a 7–8% rise in a unit's complication rate per decade of its mean age — a *group-level* (ecological) reading, not the effect of age within an individual patient (see the ecological-fallacy TRAP below)

4. The CORRELATION COEFFICIENT (r) — CRITICAL NUMBER!

r = +0.89

What 'r' means:

- **Range:** -1 to +1
- **+1:** Perfect positive correlation
- **0:** No correlation
- **-1:** Perfect negative correlation

Interpreting r = 0.89:

|r| Value	Strength	Interpretation
0.0–0.29	Weak	Little to no relationship
0.30–0.69	Moderate	Some relationship
0.70–1.00	**Strong**	**Clear relationship ← OUR DATA**

r = 0.89 = STRONG positive correlation!

5. Statistical Significance — p < 0.001

- p < 0.001: Very strong evidence against the null hypothesis of no correlation — a result this strong is extremely unlikely if there were truly no relationship.
- Less than 1 in 1,000 chance of observing a correlation this strong *if there were truly no relationship* — this is what p<0.001 means; it is not the probability that the correlation is real.
- **Statistically significant** — but always assess **clinical importance** separately (statistical significance ≠ clinical importance)

CRITICAL DISTINCTION:

- **Correlation ≠ Causation!**
- This shows age is ASSOCIATED with complications
- But doesn't prove age CAUSES complications
- Could be confounded by comorbidities, frailty, etc.

6. Scatter and Goodness of Fit

How TIGHTLY do points cluster around the line?

- **Tight clustering:** r close to ±1, line fits well, good prediction
- **Wide scatter:** r close to 0, line fits poorly, weak prediction

This plot: points lie fairly close to the line, consistent with r = 0.89

7. What to Say in Your Viva

Structure your answer like this:

Step 1 — Describe the plot:

"This scatter plot examines the relationship between mean patient age and mean complication rate across 33 surgical units — each dot is one unit."

Step 2 — Describe the pattern:

"There's a clear positive correlation — as age increases, complication rate increases. The upward-sloping regression line shows this trend."

Step 3 — Quote the correlation:

"The Pearson correlation coefficient is +0.89, indicating a strong positive correlation. This is statistically significant with p<0.001."

Step 4 — Quantify the relationship:

"Looking at the regression line, a unit with mean age 40 sits at about 5% and a unit with mean age 80 at about 35% — roughly a 7–8% higher complication rate per decade of a unit's mean age. Because this is unit-level data, I'd read it as a group-level association, not an individual-patient effect — inferring the latter would be the ecological fallacy."

Step 5 — Clinical interpretation with caution:

"At unit level, mean age is strongly associated with complication rate; individual-level prediction does not follow from it. However, correlation doesn't prove causation — age likely acts as a surrogate for accumulated comorbidities, reduced physiologic reserve, and frailty. This data supports the use of age in risk stratification models but shouldn't be used in isolation for decision-making."

⚠ COMMON EXAM TRAPS WITH SCATTER PLOTS

- **DON'T say "age causes complications"!** Say "age is associated with" or "correlates with"
- **Don't confuse correlation strength with slope:** A steep line ≠ strong correlation if points are scattered
- **Check for OUTLIERS:** One extreme point can dramatically affect the correlation
- **Linear vs non-linear:** Some relationships are curved, not straight
- **Restricted range:** Correlation only applies within the age range studied (40-80 years here)
- **Ecological fallacy:** Group-level correlation doesn't always apply to individuals
- **Confounding:** Could a third variable explain both? (Comorbidities explain age AND complications)

EXAM TIP: CORRELATION VS CAUSATION

Classic Examples to Know:

- **Ice cream sales correlate with drowning deaths** → Both caused by summer (confounding)
- **Shoe size correlates with reading ability** → Both caused by age in children

In Surgery:

- **Hospital volume correlates with outcomes** → But high-volume centres also have better resources, experienced staff, etc.
- **Drain output correlates with anastomotic leak** → Leak causes high output, not vice versa (reverse causation)

Always ask: Could there be confounding? Could causation be reversed?

QUICK EXAM-READY SUMMARY

"This scatter plot shows a strong positive correlation (r=0.89, p<0.001) between a surgical unit's mean patient age and its mean complication rate, across 33 units — roughly a 7–8% higher rate per decade of mean age. Because the data are at unit level, I'd read it as a group-level association, not an individual-patient or causal effect: age is likely a surrogate for comorbidity and reduced reserve. It supports including age in preoperative risk stratification, but not in isolation."

Chart H. ROC Curves — Diagnostic Test Performance

What you see: A curve bowing toward the top-left corner, with a diagonal reference line.
What it means: A diagnostic test's discrimination across all thresholds; the AUC is the area under it.
Key pattern: Further from the diagonal = better discrimination (AUC 0.5 = chance, nearer 1.0 = stronger). Discrimination is not the same as clinical usefulness — it doesn't replace judgement.

Viva opener: "This is an ROC curve showing a test's discrimination; the AUC summarises it, and the diagonal represents chance."

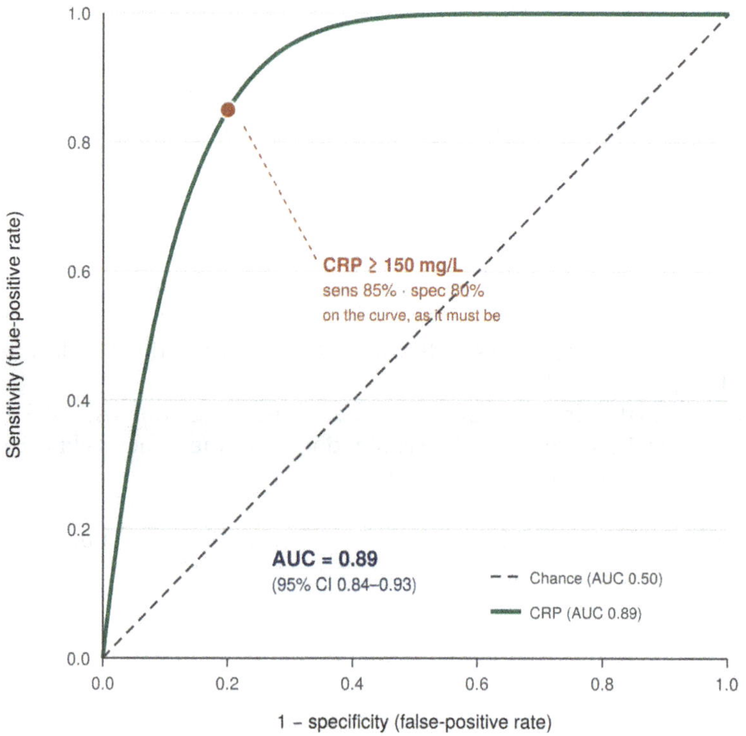

Good ranking is not the same as a trustworthy number.

Illustrative data · constructed teaching example

342 patients · every threshold of the same marker lies on this curve, so a quoted sensitivity and specificity pair must sit on it. The area says how well the marker ranks patients; it says nothing about whether the predicted risks are calibrated.

Chart H. Receiver operating characteristic curve for CRP. The curve is the locus of every threshold of the same marker, so the marked operating point lies on it: at a false-positive rate of 20% the sensitivity is 85%. The area under the curve, 0.89, measures how well the marker ranks patients and says nothing about whether the predicted risks themselves are correct. Illustrative data · a constructed teaching example, not a real study.

STUDY DETAILS:

- **Population:** 342 patients post-colorectal resection
- **Outcome:** Anastomotic leak diagnosed within 30 days
- **Test:** C-reactive protein (CRP) level on post-operative day 3
- **Result:** AUC = 0.89 indicates excellent discrimination

- **Optimal threshold:** CRP ≥150 mg/L, selected by the Youden index, which weights sensitivity and specificity equally — a cost-weighted or prespecified clinical criterion would move this cutpoint (Sensitivity 85%, Specificity 80%)

HOW TO INTERPRET ROC CURVES

1. What Are You Looking At?

A ROC (Receiver Operating Characteristic) curve shows how well a test **DISCRIMINATES** between two groups (diseased vs healthy).

- Y-AXIS: Sensitivity (true positive rate) — ability to detect disease
- X-AXIS: 1-Specificity (false positive rate) — how often test is falsely positive
- CURVE: Each point = different test threshold (cutpoint)
- DIAGONAL LINE: Random guessing (no discriminative ability)

2. Understanding the AUC (Area Under the Curve)

The single most important number on a ROC curve

AUC Value	Interpretation
1.0	Perfect test
0.90–1.00	Outstanding
0.80–0.89	Excellent
0.70–0.79	Good
0.60–0.69	Poor
0.50–0.59	Minimal discrimination

What AUC actually means: The probability that a randomly chosen patient WITH the disease scores higher than a randomly chosen patient WITHOUT the disease.

In our example: **AUC = 0.89 means** if you pick one patient with a leak and one without, there's an 89% chance the patient with the leak has a higher CRP.

3. Choosing the Optimal Cutpoint (The Marked Point)

Trade-off between sensitivity and specificity

At CRP = 150 mg/L (our optimal point):

- Sensitivity = 85%: Will detect 85% of leaks (miss 15%)
- Specificity = 80%: Will correctly identify 80% without leak (20% false alarms)

Moving the threshold UP (e.g., to 200 mg/L):

- ↓ Sensitivity (miss more leaks)

- ↑ Specificity (fewer false alarms)
- Use when: False positives are costly/harmful

Moving the threshold DOWN (e.g., to 100 mg/L):
- ↑ Sensitivity (catch more leaks)
- ↓ Specificity (more false alarms)
- Use when: Missing disease is dangerous

4. What to Say in Your Viva

Perfect structured answer:

Step 1 — Identify:
"This ROC curve evaluates CRP on post-operative day 3 as a predictor of anastomotic leak after colorectal surgery in 342 patients."

Step 2 — Interpret AUC:
"The area under the curve is 0.89 with a 95% confidence interval of 0.84 to 0.93, which indicates excellent discriminative ability. This means there's an 89% probability that a patient with an anastomotic leak will have a higher CRP than a patient without a leak."

Step 3 — Discuss optimal cutpoint:
"The optimal cutpoint is marked at 150 mg/L, where sensitivity is 85% and specificity is 80%. This means the test will identify 85% of leaks but will have a 20% false positive rate, meaning one in five patients without a leak will be flagged."

Step 4 — Clinical application:
"Clinically, this suggests that a CRP of 150 mg/L or above on day 3 should prompt consideration of anastomotic leak, possibly triggering a CT scan with oral contrast or closer monitoring. However, we must balance sensitivity against the resource implications of investigating 20% false positives. In practice, I would use this as part of a clinical scoring system, not as a standalone diagnostic test."

⚠ COMMON PITFALLS AND EXAMINER TRAPS

- **DON'T confuse AUC with accuracy:** AUC measures discrimination, not overall accuracy
- **DON'T assume AUC >0.7 means clinically useful:** Depends on disease prevalence and consequences
- **DON'T forget confidence intervals:** Wide CIs mean uncertainty
- **DON'T apply cutpoints blindly:** Optimal point depends on clinical context
- **DO remember:** A perfect AUC (1.0) suggests overfitting or data problems

Clinical Applications of ROC Curves in Surgery

- **Risk prediction models:** POSSUM score for predicting mortality (AUC ~0.8)

- **Biomarkers:** CRP, procalcitonin for predicting complications
- **Imaging:** CT findings for predicting malignancy
- **Scoring systems:** Glasgow-Blatchford score for GI bleeding
- **Genomic tests:** Oncotype DX for predicting chemotherapy benefit

Remember: ROC curves don't tell you if a test is clinically useful — they only tell you how well it discriminates. A test with AUC 0.95 might still be useless if it's too expensive, too invasive, or doesn't change management.

WHAT EXAMINERS REWARD

When shown a ROC curve, most candidates just quote the AUC. **The best answers go further.** Discuss what threshold you'd actually use in practice — would you prioritise sensitivity (catching all leaks, accepting false alarms) or specificity (avoiding unnecessary investigations)? For anastomotic leak, I'd argue for high sensitivity because missing a leak is catastrophic, whereas a false positive just means an extra CT scan.

Also mention: ROC curves assume disease prevalence doesn't matter, but it does clinically. If leak rate is 5%, even a test with 85% sensitivity and 80% specificity will have lots of false positives. Calculate positive predictive value to show you understand this.

QUICK EXAM-READY SUMMARY

Perfect 45-second response:

"This ROC curve evaluates C-reactive protein on post-operative day 3 as a predictor of anastomotic leak. The AUC of 0.89 with 95% CI 0.84-0.93 indicates excellent discriminative ability — there's an 89% chance a patient with a leak has a higher CRP than one without. The optimal cutpoint at 150 mg/L gives 85% sensitivity and 80% specificity. Clinically, this could be useful as a screening tool to identify high-risk patients requiring closer monitoring or CT imaging, though the 20% false positive rate means we couldn't use it alone as a diagnostic test. The high AUC suggests CRP is a valuable biomarker that should be incorporated into clinical decision algorithms for early leak detection."

Chart I. Funnel Plots — Publication Bias in Meta-Analysis

What you see: A scattered cloud of dots in a rough inverted-funnel shape, widest at the bottom.

What it means: A check for publication bias in a meta-analysis: effect size (x-axis) against precision (y-axis).

Key pattern: Symmetry is reassuring; a gap (usually a bottom corner) suggests possible publication bias — but asymmetry has other causes, and you need roughly ten studies before interpreting it.

Viva opener: "This is a funnel plot assessing publication bias; I'd look for asymmetry, while noting it has several causes and needs about ten studies to interpret."

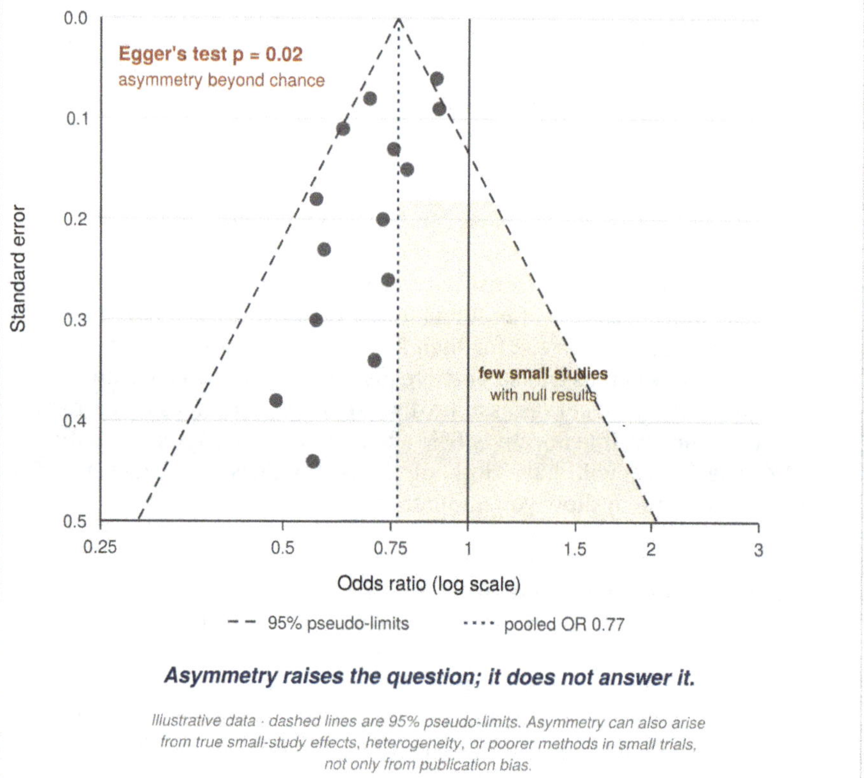

Chart I. Publication-bias funnel plot, with standard error on an inverted vertical axis so the 95% pseudo-limits are straight lines. Fourteen studies pool to an odds ratio of 0.77. Large studies cluster near the pooled estimate; smaller studies scatter only to the left, and the shaded region shows where small studies with null results would sit if they existed. Egger's test gives p = 0.02.

⚠ WARNING: FUNNEL-PLOT ASYMMETRY DETECTED!

- **Asymmetry observed:** Small studies on the right (OR>1, unfavourable to laparoscopic / favouring open surgery) are missing

- **Egger's test:** $p = 0.02$ (significant asymmetry)
- Trim-and-fill analysis: imputes 7 studies (L0 estimator) on the under-represented right-hand side; the R0 estimator is unstable here, and different implementations disagree
- **Implication:** The pooled benefit of laparoscopic surgery may be overestimated
- Adjusted estimate: if the asymmetry reflects suppression, filling those 7 studies moves the pooled OR from 0.77 to about 0.85 — towards the null, and still favouring laparoscopic surgery

HOW TO INTERPRET FUNNEL PLOTS

1. What Are You Looking At?

A funnel plot is a **SCATTER PLOT** used to detect publication bias in meta-analyses.

- **X-AXIS:** Effect size (Odds Ratio, Risk Ratio, Mean Difference)
- **Y-AXIS:** Study precision (usually Standard Error — inverted so large studies are at top)
- **EACH DOT:** One study in the meta-analysis
- **FUNNEL SHAPE:** Expected distribution if no publication bias

Why it's shaped like a funnel:

- **Top (large studies):** High precision, tightly clustered near true effect
- **Bottom (small studies):** Low precision, widely scattered due to sampling error
- **If no bias:** Studies should be symmetrically distributed around the true effect

2. What Is Publication Bias?

The problem: Studies with negative or null results are less likely to be published than positive studies.

Why does it happen?

- **Journals prefer novelty:** "Dog bites man" (expected result) doesn't get published; "Man bites dog" (surprising result) does
- **Authors don't submit:** Negative results sit in "file drawers" unpublished
- **Industry suppression:** Drug companies may not publish unfavourable trials
- **Confirmation bias:** Researchers pursue positive findings, abandon negative ones

Why does it matter?

If only positive studies are published, meta-analyses will **OVERESTIMATE** treatment effects. A drug that looks miraculous might actually be mediocre once missing negative studies are accounted for.

3. Reading the Asymmetry — Is There Bias?

✓ **SYMMETRIC FUNNEL = NO BIAS**

What you see:

- Studies evenly distributed on both sides
- Perfect inverted funnel shape
- Small studies scattered but centred

Interpretation: No evidence of publication bias. Meta-analysis result is likely reliable.

X ASYMMETRIC FUNNEL = BIAS SUSPECTED

What you see:

- Missing studies on one side (usually bottom-right for OR-based plots)
- Gap in bottom-right corner
- Lopsided distribution

Interpretation: Publication bias likely. True effect is probably smaller than meta-analysis suggests.

In our example:

The bottom-right corner is nearly empty — small studies with OR>1 (unfavourable to laparoscopic / favouring open surgery) are missing. This suggests that unfavourable laparoscopic results were not published, inflating the apparent benefit of laparoscopic surgery.

4. Statistical Tests for Publication Bias

Test	What It Does	Interpretation
Egger's test	Statistical test for asymmetry	p<0.05 = significant asymmetry
Begg's test	Rank correlation test	Less powerful than Egger's
Trim-and-fill	Estimates missing studies & adjusts pooled effect	Shows what result would be if bias corrected

In our example: Egger's test gives p=0.02, which is statistical evidence of the same asymmetry — supporting the visual impression rather than independently confirming it, since both readings come from the same data, and noting that the test has limited power with as few as fourteen studies. Trim-and-fill imputes 7 missing studies and moves the pooled OR from 0.77 to approximately 0.85. Treat that as a sensitivity analysis rather than a corrected result: 7 imputed studies against 14 observed means a third of the filled dataset is invented, and the adjusted confidence interval ignores that.

5. What to Say in Your Viva

Perfect structured answer:

Step 1 — Identify:

"This funnel plot displays 14 randomised controlled trials comparing laparoscopic versus open colorectal surgery. Each dot represents one trial, plotted by effect size (odds ratio) on the x-axis and precision (standard error, inverted) on the y-axis, so the most precise trials sit at the top."

Step 2 — Assess symmetry:

"There is clear asymmetry — the bottom-right corner is notably sparse. Small studies showing results unfavourable to laparoscopic (OR>1) appear to be missing, while small positive studies favouring laparoscopic surgery are present."

Step 3 — Statistical confirmation:

"Egger's test supports this with p=0.02, indicating statistically significant funnel-plot asymmetry, of which publication bias is one possible cause. Trim-and-fill imputes 7 missing studies and moves the pooled odds ratio from 0.77 to roughly 0.85 — towards the null, though that adjustment assumes the asymmetry is entirely due to suppression."

Step 4 — Clinical interpretation:

"This suggests the meta-analysis likely overestimates the benefit of laparoscopic surgery. Laparoscopic surgery still shows benefit after adjustment, at an odds ratio of about 0.85 rather than 0.77, so the true effect is probably more modest than the published literature suggests. This highlights the importance of trial registration and mandatory publication of all results to prevent bias."

Step 5 — Limitations:

"However, asymmetry doesn't always mean publication bias — it could also reflect true heterogeneity, differences in methodological quality, or chance. I would want to examine if there's a relationship between study quality and effect size before concluding definitively."

⚠ Other Causes of Funnel Plot Asymmetry (Not Just Publication Bias!)

- **Heterogeneity:** Small studies done in different populations (e.g., sicker patients) may have genuinely different effects
- **Poor methodological quality:** Small studies often have weaker methods, leading to inflated effects
- **Language bias:** Non-English studies may have different results
- **Chance:** With <10 studies, asymmetry can occur randomly
- **True early benefit:** Early small studies might show larger effects if learning curve improves over time

⚠ **CRITICAL EXAMINER POINT:** Don't automatically assume asymmetry = publication bias. Always consider alternative explanations and check if patterns relate to study quality, publication year, or patient characteristics.

Preventing Publication Bias — What You Can Do

1. **Trial registration:** Register trials prospectively (ClinicalTrials.gov, ISRCTN)

2. **Mandatory reporting:** Journals require registration before enrolment starts
3. **Search unpublished data:** Contact authors, search conference abstracts, check trial registries
4. **Protocol publication:** Publish study protocol before results known
5. **Open science:** Pre-register analysis plans, share data publicly

WHAT EXAMINERS REWARD

Funnel plots are a favourite because they reveal if candidates understand meta-analysis limitations. **The best answers acknowledge publication bias but also mention alternative explanations.** Don't just say 'there's bias' — explain what trim-and-fill tells you, and whether the adjusted result still changes practice. For our example, adjustment moves the odds ratio from 0.77 to about 0.85 — laparoscopic surgery still shows benefit, but the magnitude matters for cost-effectiveness and patient counselling. **Also key:** Mention prospective trial registration as the solution. Show you understand how modern research practices prevent publication bias rather than just detecting it after the fact.

QUICK EXAM-READY SUMMARY

Perfect 60-second response:

"This funnel plot examines publication bias in a meta-analysis of 14 RCTs comparing laparoscopic versus open colorectal surgery. The plot shows clear asymmetry with a sparse bottom-right corner, indicating missing small studies unfavourable to laparoscopic surgery (OR>1, favouring open).

Egger's test supports this with p=0.02. If the asymmetry reflects missing studies, adjustment would move the pooled estimate closer to the null, suggesting the published literature may overstate the benefit of laparoscopic surgery. Trim-and-fill imputes 7 studies and shifts the pooled odds ratio from 0.77 to about 0.85; a benefit survives, but with a third of the filled dataset imputed this is a sensitivity analysis, not a corrected answer.

This asymmetry could reflect true publication bias but might also indicate heterogeneity or methodological differences. The solution is prospective trial registration and mandatory publication of all results.

Clinically, this tells us to interpret meta-analyses cautiously and consider that real-world benefits may be more modest than reported."

Chart J. CONSORT Flow Diagram — Where Patients Are Lost

What you see: A vertical cascade of boxes, starting with everyone screened and narrowing to the numbers finally analysed, with side boxes for those excluded or lost.

What it means: The audit trail of an RCT: it accounts for every patient from first contact to final analysis.

Key pattern: Read it *bottom-up*. If the number analysed is smaller than the number randomised, ask why. Without imputation this is usually a complete-case or modified intention-to-treat analysis rather than a true intention-to-treat — whatever the paper calls it.
Viva opener: "This is the CONSORT flow diagram. I'd start at the bottom and check whether everyone randomised was analysed, then look at attrition in each arm."

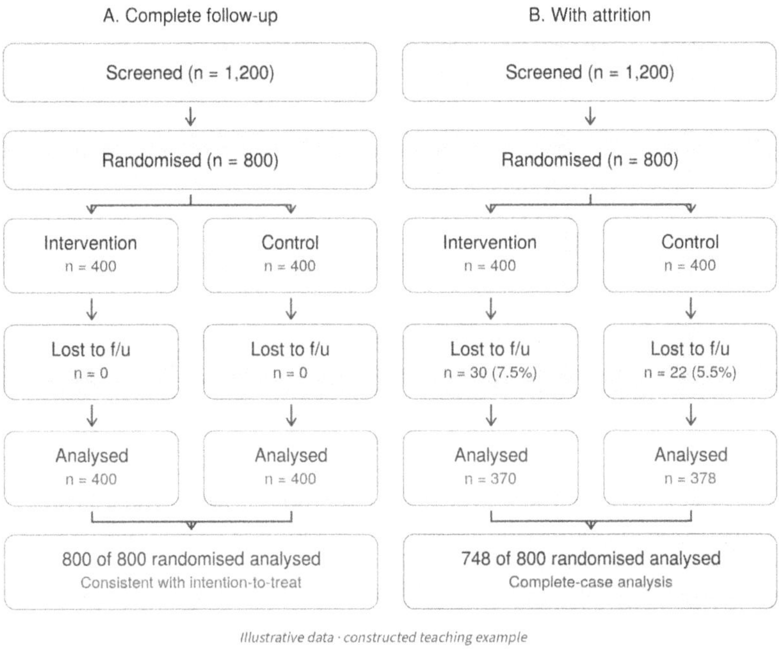

Chart J. CONSORT flow diagrams compared. Panel A: all 800 randomised participants are analysed in their allocated groups, consistent with the intention-to-treat principle. Panel B: 30 participants are lost from the intervention arm and 22 from control, leaving 748 analysed — a complete-case analysis unless the authors imputed missing outcome data. Illustrative data · a constructed teaching example, not a real study.

READING A CONSORT DIAGRAM IN THE VIVA

- **Screened → randomised.** A steep drop (here 1,200 to 800) signals a highly selected population. It does not invalidate the trial, but it does limit who the result applies to.

- **Randomised → received allocation.** Patients who never received their allocated treatment still belong to their original group under ITT. This is where crossover hides.
- **Attrition.** Loss to follow-up above roughly 20%, or clearly unequal between arms, threatens validity — and unequal loss is the more serious of the two, because it suggests the reason for leaving is related to treatment.
- **Analysed vs randomised.** The single most useful comparison on the page.

⚠ THE COMMONEST ERROR

Candidates describe the diagram instead of interrogating it. Do not read the numbers aloud — the examiner can see them. Say what they *mean*: "Thirty patients were lost from the intervention arm against twenty-two from control, and since only 748 of the 800 randomised are analysed, this is a complete-case analysis, not a true intention-to-treat analysis."

Chart K. PRISMA Flow Diagram — How a Review Was Assembled

What you see: A funnel of records: thousands identified, narrowing through de-duplication and screening to the handful of studies finally pooled.

What it means: The search and selection audit trail of a systematic review or meta-analysis.

Key pattern: Judge the *breadth of the search* at the top and the *transparency of exclusions* at the bottom. Full-text exclusions must be counted with reasons.

Viva opener: "This is the PRISMA flow diagram. I'd want to know how wide the search was, and whether the full-text exclusions were reported with reasons."

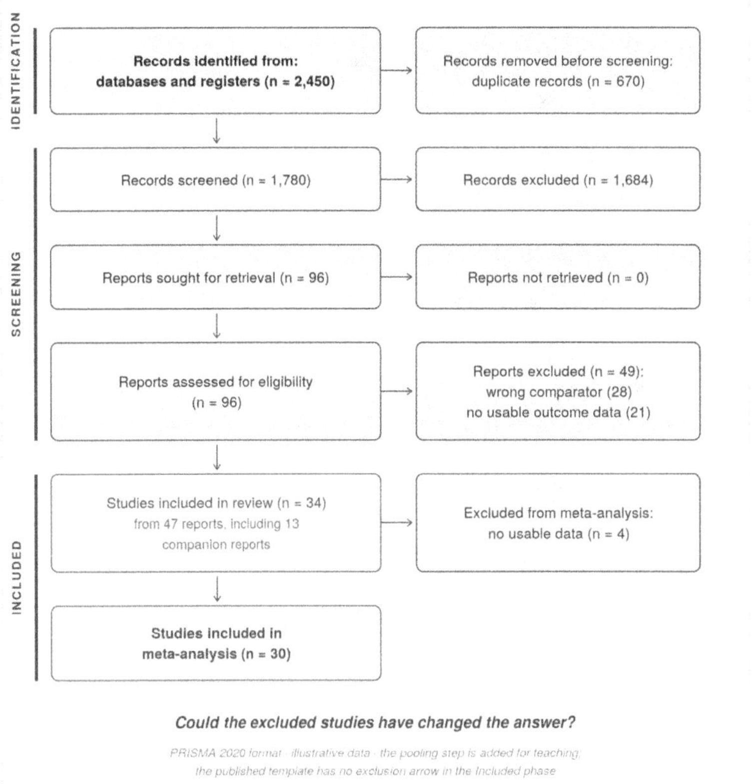

Chart K. PRISMA 2020 flow diagram. Records are search hits, reports are documents, and studies are the unit of analysis: 47 reports remained after full-text exclusion, but these described only 34 studies because 13 were companion reports of studies already counted. Four of those 34 could not be pooled, leaving 30 in the meta-analysis.

WHAT THE PRISMA DIAGRAM TELLS YOU

- **Search breadth.** One database, no grey literature, English-only — each narrows the evidence base and feeds the publication bias you would assess on the funnel plot (Chart I).
- **Screening attrition is normal.** Dropping 1,780 records to 96 full texts is not a criticism; that is what screening is for.
- **Full-text exclusions are where the judgement lies.** These must be listed with reasons. Vague or absent reasons here are a legitimate criticism.

- **Included in synthesis vs meta-analysis.** Studies included in the review but excluded from pooling (here 34 versus 30) are easy to miss and often the ones with unusable or divergent data.

LINKING THE THREE META-ANALYSIS CHARTS

PRISMA (Chart K) tells you *which* studies were pooled, the forest plot (Chart B) tells you *what* they showed and how consistent they were, and the funnel plot (Chart I) asks whether the ones you can see are the whole story. A strong candidate moves between all three.

Chart L. Cumulative Incidence — Competing Risks

What you see: Curves rising from zero, often with a second curve for the competing event, and frequently a higher Kaplan–Meier curve drawn alongside for comparison.

What it means: The probability of experiencing the event of interest over time when other events can prevent it from ever happening.

Key pattern: The gap between the naive Kaplan–Meier curve and the cumulative incidence function *widens with follow-up*, and widens fastest in elderly or comorbid cohorts.

Viva opener: "This is a cumulative incidence curve accounting for competing risks — appropriate here, because death from other causes prevents the recurrence we are measuring."

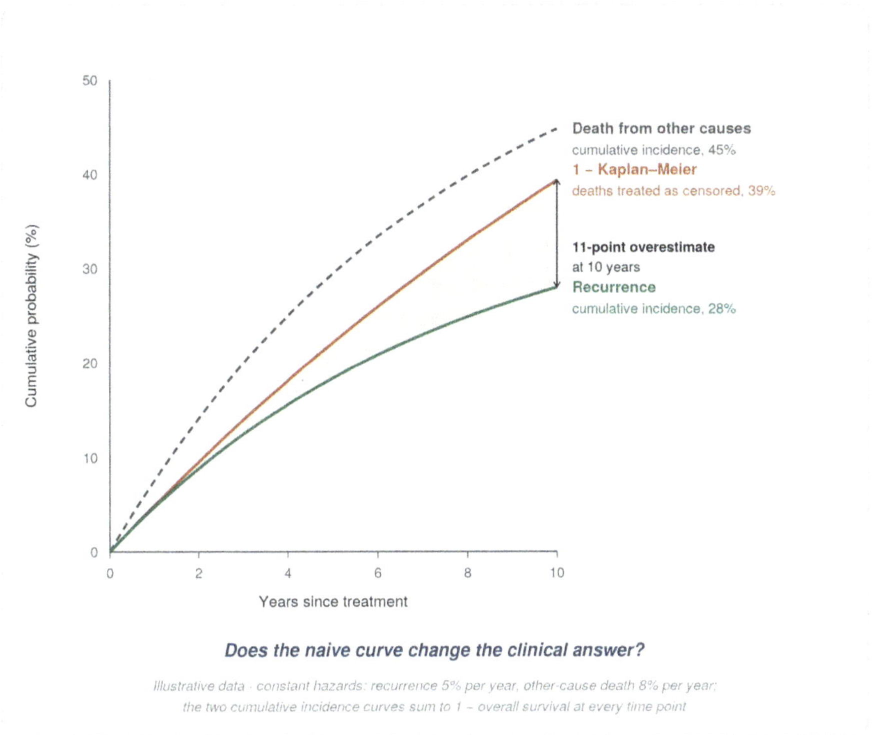

Chart L. Cumulative incidence with competing risks. Treating other-cause deaths as censored assumes those patients could still recur, so 1 – Kaplan–Meier lies above the cumulative incidence function whenever any competing event occurs, and the shaded gap widens with follow-up. The two cumulative incidence curves sum to 1 – overall survival at every time point.

WHY THE TWO CURVES DIVERGE

Kaplan–Meier treats a competing death as *censored*, which assumes the patient could still have had the event later. They could not. That assumption inflates the estimate, and the inflation compounds over time — which is exactly why the gap in the figure grows with follow-up rather than staying constant.

- **Use the CIF** whenever a competing event is common: elderly cohorts, long follow-up, cancer studies reporting recurrence rather than death.
- **Fine–Gray regression** models the subdistribution hazard, which is a related but distinct question from cause-specific hazards.
- **The give-away** is a paper reporting "freedom from recurrence" by Kaplan–Meier in a population with substantial non-cancer mortality.

WHAT EXAMINERS REWARD

Competing risks is where good candidates separate themselves. Anyone can recite what a Kaplan–Meier curve shows. The candidate who looks at an eighty-year-old cohort and asks whether death from other causes was handled properly is thinking like someone who will interpret evidence for the rest of their career.

Chart M. Calibration Plot — Do Predicted Risks Match Reality?

What you see: Predicted risk on the x-axis against observed risk on the y-axis, with a 45° reference line and either grouped observations (for example, deciles of predicted risk) or a flexible calibration curve.
What it means: Whether a risk model's numbers are *true*. If it says 20%, do 20 in 100 actually have the event?
Key pattern: Points on the diagonal = well calibrated. Below it = the model over-predicts; above it = it under-predicts. Deviation typically worsens at the extremes of risk.
Viva opener: "This is a calibration plot. The AUC tells me the model ranks patients well, but this tells me whether the actual risk figures can be trusted at the bedside."

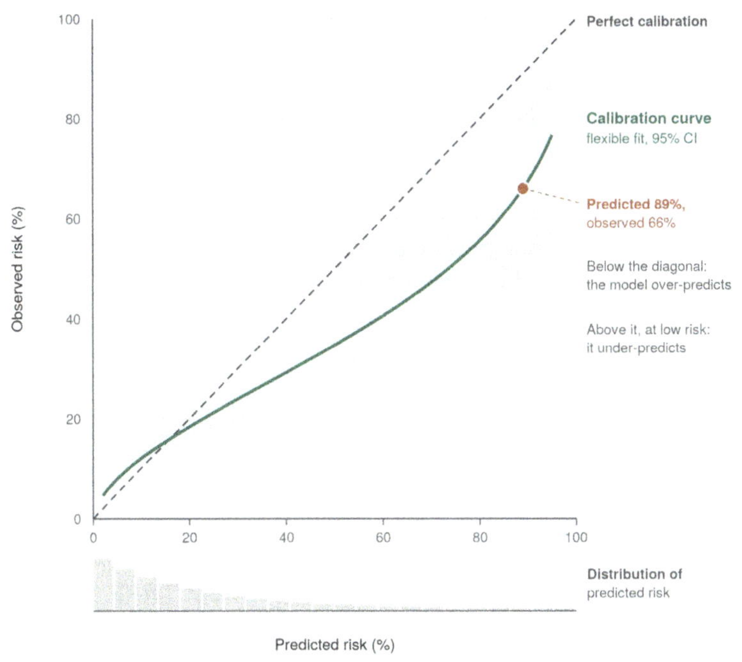

Would you quote this number in a consent conversation?

Illustrative data logistic recalibration with slope 0.62; the curve crosses the diagonal at 16%, and the confidence limits widen where few patients sit

Chart M. Calibration plot with a flexible calibration curve rather than decile groupings. A calibration slope below 1 makes predictions too extreme, so high predictions run too high and low predictions too low. In this constructed example the curve crosses the ideal line at about 16%, and the model quotes 89% where the observed rate is 66%. The crossing point depends on the intercept as well as the slope, so it is specific to this figure rather than a general consequence of a slope below 1. The histogram shows how few patients sit at high predicted risk, which is why the confidence limits widen there. Discrimination is unaffected by miscalibration — rescaling predictions leaves the ranking, and therefore the AUC, unchanged.

Discrimination and calibration are different things

A model can rank patients perfectly and still produce numbers that are wrong. Discrimination (the AUC, Chart H) asks *does it put the higher-risk patient above the lower-risk one?* Calibration asks *is 20% really 20%?* The model plotted here has an AUC of 0.81 — respectable — yet tells a patient their risk is 89% when the observed rate is 66%.

- **Why it matters clinically.** Consent, prehabilitation and critical-care planning all use the absolute number, not the ranking. An over-predicting model frightens patients and over-books intensive care.
- **Calibration-in-the-large** is whether average predicted risk matches average observed risk; the **calibration slope** is whether predictions are too extreme (slope < 1) or too flat.
- **The Hosmer–Lemeshow test** is often quoted here. Treat it cautiously: it is underpowered in small samples and rejects almost any model in very large ones. The plot is more informative than its p-value.
- **Calibration drifts** as case-mix and practice change, which is why models such as P-POSSUM and NELA need periodic recalibration rather than permanent trust.

WHAT EXAMINERS REWARD

If a candidate tells me a risk model has an AUC of 0.8 and stops there, I ask whether it is calibrated. Most cannot answer. It is the difference between a model that sorts patients and a model you can quote a number from in a consent conversation.

Chart N. Subgroup Forest Plot — The Commonest TRAP

What you see: The overall trial result at the top, then the same result split by age, sex, stage, approach and so on — each with its own estimate and confidence interval.

What it means: An exploration of whether the treatment effect differs between groups. It is *hypothesis-generating*, not confirmatory.

Key pattern: Ignore which subgroups reached significance. Look for the **test for interaction** — that is the only legitimate test of whether the effect truly differs. Note the converse: interaction tests are often underpowered, so a non-significant interaction does not prove the effect is the same across subgroups — only that the trial could not detect a difference.

Viva opener: "This is a subgroup analysis. Before interpreting any individual subgroup I'd want the test for interaction, and I'd want to know whether these subgroups were pre-specified."

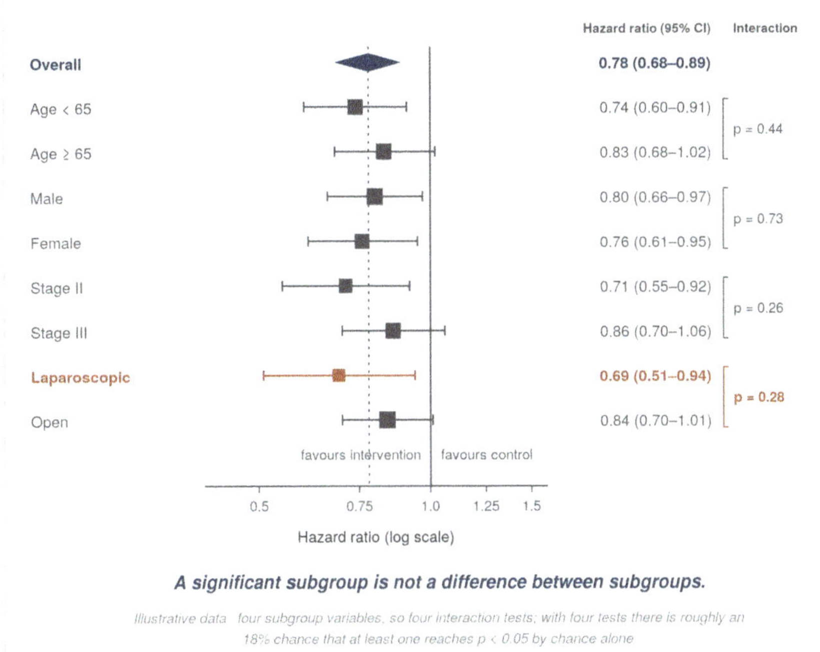

Chart N. Subgroup forest plot. Eight subgroup rows come from four subgroup variables, so there are four interaction tests, not eight. The laparoscopic subgroup reaches significance (HR 0.69, p = 0.02) and the open subgroup does not (p = 0.06), yet the test for interaction is p = 0.28: there is no evidence the effect differs by approach. Marker size is proportional to precision, and the vertical dotted line marks the overall estimate.

⚠ THE TRAP, AND HOW TO AVOID IT

In the figure, the laparoscopic subgroup reaches significance (HR 0.69, p=0.02) while the open subgroup does not. The tempting conclusion — “the treatment works in laparoscopic patients” — is wrong, and naming why is what scores.

- **The interaction test is p=0.28.** There is no evidence the effect genuinely differs between approaches. A significant result in one subgroup and not another is *not* evidence of a difference between them.
- **Multiplicity.** Test enough subgroups at p<0.05 and roughly one in twenty will be “significant” by chance alone. With four interaction tests, a spurious result is a real possibility.

- **Power.** Each subgroup is a fraction of the trial, so confidence intervals widen and non-significance usually reflects lost power, not absent effect.
- **Pre-specified or post-hoc?** Pre-specified subgroups with a stated interaction test carry some weight. Post-hoc subgroups are exploratory, whatever the p-value.
- **The best estimate for any individual subgroup** is usually the overall result, not that subgroup's own estimate.

THE SENTENCE THAT SCORES

"The laparoscopic subgroup appears to benefit more, but the test for interaction is non-significant at p=0.28, so I would not conclude the effect differs by approach. With four interaction tests — eight rows, but only four subgroup variables — an apparently significant result could still arise by chance. I would treat this as hypothesis-generating and apply the overall estimate to all patients."

Chart O. Institutional Funnel Plot — Outcome Monitoring

What you see: Each unit or surgeon plotted as a dot: case volume on the x-axis, risk-adjusted outcome on the y-axis, inside curved control limits that narrow as volume rises.

What it means: Whether any unit's results differ from the national average by more than chance would explain. This is **outcome monitoring, not publication bias** — a different chart entirely from Chart I.

Key pattern: The funnel narrows with volume because small units have genuinely more uncertain estimates. A dot outside the 99.8% limits is a signal to investigate, not a verdict.

Viva opener: "This is an institutional funnel plot used for outcome monitoring. I'd check the risk adjustment first, then look for units outside the 99.8% limits."

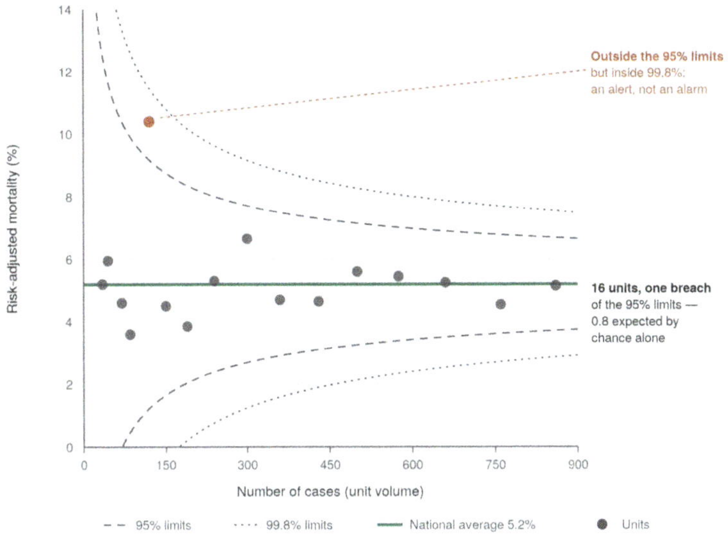

An outlier is a question, not a verdict.

Illustrative data · binomial limits around a national average of 5.2%, with no adjustment for overdispersion; below about 70 cases the lower 95% limit reaches zero, so a small unit cannot be flagged as good

Chart O. Institutional funnel plot. The limits narrow with volume because larger units have more precise estimates. One unit of sixteen lies outside the 95% limits and inside the 99.8% limits — an alert rather than an alarm, and close to the 0.8 breaches expected by chance alone when sixteen units are plotted. Limits here are binomial only; real audit data are usually overdispersed, and unadjusted limits flag too many units.

HOW TO APPRAISE ONE PROPERLY

- **Risk adjustment is everything.** A unit taking the sickest patients will look worse unless the model adjusts adequately — and the adjustment model itself needs calibrating (Chart M).
- **Alert and alarm.** Outside 95% is conventionally an alert, outside 99.8% an alarm. With many units, some will breach the 95% limits by chance alone.
- **Never rank into a league table.** Ranks are far less stable than they appear; units in the middle are statistically indistinguishable from one another.
- **Regression to the mean.** A unit flagged one year often returns towards average the next without any change in practice.
- **An outlier is a question, not an answer.** The correct response is investigation — data quality first, then case-mix, then process.

Chart P. Bland–Altman Plots — Agreement, Not Correlation

What you see: A scatter of one point per patient, plotting the difference between two measurements against their mean. A central horizontal line and two outer horizontal lines.

What it means: Whether two methods, observers or devices can be used interchangeably. The central line is the mean difference — systematic bias. The outer lines are the 95% limits of agreement, mean difference ± 1.96 SD of the differences.

Key pattern: Read the width of the limits, not the scatter of the points. The question is never whether most points lie inside the limits — by construction about 95% will. The question is whether that range of disagreement is clinically tolerable.

Viva opener: "This is a Bland–Altman plot assessing agreement between two measurement methods. The central line is the mean difference, or systematic bias, and the outer lines are the 95% limits of agreement. I would look for fixed bias, proportional bias, outliers, and above all whether those limits are clinically acceptable."

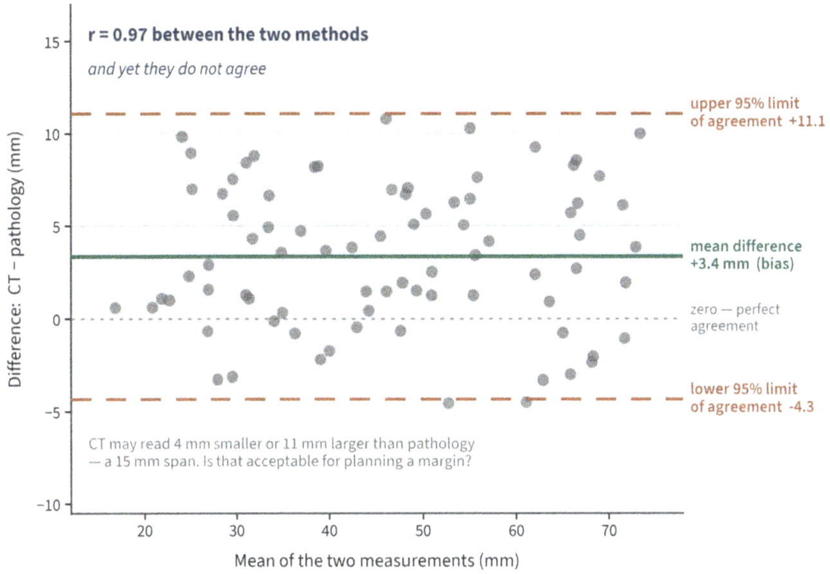

Correlation is not agreement.

Illustrative data · 80 patients, CT versus pathological tumour diameter. The limits of agreement are mean difference ± 1.96 SD of the differences; they describe where 95% of individual disagreements fall. Whether that range is acceptable is a clinical judgement, not a statistical one.

Chart P. Agreement between CT and pathological tumour diameter in 80 patients. The two methods correlate at r = 0.97, yet CT reads on average 3.4 mm larger than pathology, and the 95% limits of agreement run from −4.3 mm to +11.1 mm. An individual CT may therefore read 4 mm smaller or 11 mm larger than the true diameter — a 15 mm span. There is no proportional bias (slope +0.004 mm per mm, p = 0.88), so the limits apply across the measured range. Correlation measures whether values move together; agreement measures whether they are the same.

Why correlation fails here

A correlation coefficient asks whether two measurements rise and fall together. Two methods can do that perfectly while one reads consistently 10 mm high. Multiply every pathology measurement by two and the correlation does not move — a perfect 1.00 stays 1.00 — though the methods now agree nowhere at all.

Correlation is also inflated by a wide measurement range: study tumours from 5 mm to 200 mm and r will look excellent whatever the disagreement, because between-patient variation swamps between-method variation.

What to look for

Fixed bias. The central line sits away from zero: one method reads consistently high or low. This is often correctable by calibration.

Proportional bias. The points slope upward or downward across the plot, so disagreement changes with the size of the measurement. The ordinary limits are then misleading.

Heteroscedasticity. The scatter fans out to the right: variability grows with magnitude, and a log transformation may be needed.

Outliers. Isolated extreme differences — ask whether these are measurement failures or real cases.

Repeated measurements. Ordinary Bland–Altman assumes one pair per subject; if patients contribute more than one pair, the within-subject dependence must be handled.

Normality of the differences. The ±1.96 SD construction only delivers 95% coverage if the differences are approximately normal. In this example they are (Shapiro–Wilk $p = 0.13$), but the assumption should be checked rather than assumed.

The clinical judgement

The limits of agreement are a description, not a verdict. Whether that 15 mm span matters depends entirely on what the measurement is used for. For deciding a resection margin it may be decisive; for gross staging it may not. An examiner is asking whether you can connect a statistical interval to a clinical decision — that is the whole point of the plot.

Note also that the limits themselves are estimates. Each limit has a standard error of about SD × the square root of 3/n, so with 80 patients each carries a 95% confidence interval of roughly ±1.5 mm: the upper limit of +11.1 mm is really 9.6 to 12.6 mm, and the mean difference of +3.4 mm is 2.5 to 4.3 mm. A small study estimates its limits imprecisely, so their own confidence intervals are wide, and an apparently narrow observed spread may not represent the population — always ask how many patients produced them.

One further point for the pedantic examiner: pathology here is close to a reference standard, and where one method is a gold standard some authors plot the difference against that reference rather than against the mean. Bland and Altman argued for the mean because it assumes both methods are measured with error, which is usually the safer assumption.

Common Exam Error: agreement is not "most points inside the limits"

Saying the methods agree because they correlate, or because most points lie between the limits. Both miss the point — about 95% of points fall inside the limits by construction, however bad the agreement is. Say what the limits mean in millimetres, then say whether that range is acceptable for the clinical purpose. Do not say that the methods correlate well so they agree, that most points lie within the limits so the methods are interchangeable, that the limits are statistically significant, or that a narrow confidence interval around the mean difference proves good agreement.

60-second model answer

"This Bland–Altman plot assesses agreement between CT and pathological measurement of tumour diameter in 80 patients. There is a fixed bias of 3.4 mm, with CT reading larger, and the 95% limits of agreement run from −4.3 to +11.1 mm. So although the two methods correlate at 0.97, an individual CT measurement could be 4 mm below or 11 mm above the pathological diameter. I would not treat these as interchangeable for decisions sensitive to a centimetre, such as margin planning, though the bias is systematic and might be correctable. These limits are themselves estimates: with 80 patients each carries a 95% confidence interval of about 1.5 mm either way, so the upper limit of 11.1 mm is really between 9.6 and 12.6 mm. I would also want to know whether measurements were paired one per patient, whether observers were blinded to each other, and whether the spread widens with tumour size, since that would make the limits misleading."

Examiner Follow-Up: "The upper limit could be as high as 12.6 mm. Does that change your interpretation?"
Answer: "It does not change the qualitative conclusion — a 12.6 mm upper limit is still clinically meaningful for margin planning. But it is a reminder that the limits are estimates, not fixed boundaries. I would want to know the sample size: with 80 patients the precision is reasonable, but with 20 patients the limits would be far less reliable."

For categorical agreement

Bland–Altman applies to continuous measurements. Where two observers assign categories — a scan reported as positive or negative — agreement is assessed with Cohen's kappa, which corrects for agreement expected by chance. A raw percentage agreement figure is not sufficient, because two observers who both call almost everything negative will agree most of the time by chance alone. Where the categories are ordered, such as tumour grade I to IV, use weighted kappa: plain kappa treats a grade I versus IV disagreement as no worse than I versus II.

ADVANCED CONTENT MODULES

Go Beyond the Basics: Master Complex Concepts for Excellence
These enrichment modules provide advanced statistical concepts, complex study designs, and detailed clinical scenarios with model viva answers to transform you from a competent candidate into an outstanding one.

MODULE 1: Advanced Clinical Chart Examples

Six detailed surgical scenarios (Examples 1-6) covering grouped bar charts, scatter plots, pie charts, box plots, ROC curves, and funnel plots. Each includes 5-second recognition drills, step-by-step interpretation, model viva responses, and common examiner follow-ups.

UPPER GI SURGERY

Example 1: Grouped Bar Chart — Anastomotic Leak Risk Factors

Clinical Scenario:

Multi-centre cohort study of 1,847 patients undergoing oesophagectomy. Investigators examined modifiable risk factors for anastomotic leak. Results presented as grouped bar chart comparing leak rates across smoking status, diabetes control, and BMI categories.

Anastomotic Leak Rates by Risk Factor Category

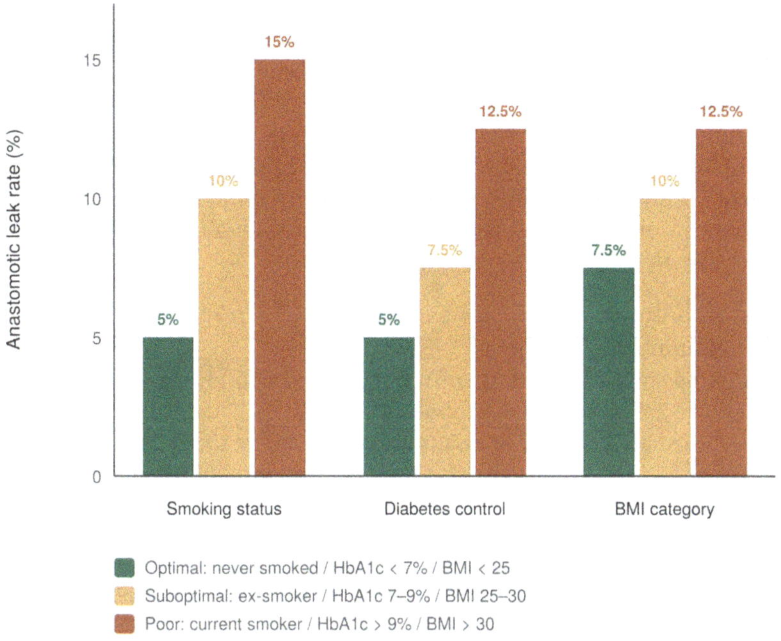

Illustrative data · 1,847 patients. Rates are marginal, so a patient with all three risk factors is counted in all three groups; a combined risk needs a multivariable model.

5-SECOND RECOGNITION DRILL

What you see: Three groups of coloured bars, each group showing progression from low → intermediate → high risk

What it means: Comparing risk across categories of modifiable factors

Key pattern: Consistent gradient — worse control = higher leak rate across all three factors

Viva opener: "This grouped bar chart demonstrates dose-response relationships between three modifiable risk factors and anastomotic leak rates"

Step-by-Step Interpretation

1. Identify the Pattern

- **Consistent trend:** All three factors show linear increase in leak risk
- **Smoking:** 3-fold increase (5% → 15%)

- **Diabetes:** 2.5-fold increase (5% → 12.5%)
- **BMI:** 1.7-fold increase (7.5% → 12.5%)

2. Calculate Absolute and Relative Risk

Smoking (Optimal vs Poor):

- ARR = 15% - 5% = 10%
- Relative risk = 15% / 5% = 3.0; the relative difference is 67% of the smokers' risk. This is an association between exposure groups, not the effect of quitting.
- Absolute risk increase = 10 percentage points, or roughly one extra leak for every 10 patients in the higher-risk group. This is an observational comparison between exposure groups, not an intervention effect, so it is better described as an absolute risk increase than as a number needed to harm.

3. Assess Clinical Significance

Which factor matters most?

- Smoking shows **largest absolute effect** (10% difference)
- All three are modifiable preoperatively
- Combined effect: these are marginal rates, so the three cannot simply be added — estimating the risk for a patient with all three needs a multivariable model

PERFECT 60-SECOND MODEL VIVA RESPONSE

"This grouped bar chart from a cohort of 1,847 oesophagectomy patients demonstrates dose-response relationships between three modifiable risk factors and anastomotic leak rates.

The pattern is consistent across all three factors — poorer control correlates with higher leak rates. Smoking shows the most dramatic effect: current smokers have a 15% leak rate versus 5% in never-smokers, representing an absolute risk increase of 10% and a 3-fold relative risk. This means one additional leak occurs for every 10 current smokers operated on.

Diabetes control and BMI show similar but less pronounced gradients. Importantly, these are all potentially modifiable factors. Clinically, this data supports preoperative optimisation — cessation support, glycaemic optimisation and attention to nutritional state. What it cannot tell us is how much of the difference between exposure groups would be recovered by changing the exposure.

The limitation is that this is observational data — we can't prove causation. Patients who smoke may have other unmeasured confounders like poor nutrition or comorbidities. However, the consistent biological plausibility and dose-response relationship strengthen the argument for preoperative intervention programmes."

⚠ COMMON EXAMINER FOLLOW-UPS & HOW TO ANSWER

Q: "These are all modifiable — would you delay surgery to optimise?"
A: "It depends on cancer stage. For locally advanced cancers, neoadjuvant therapy provides a 6-8 week window for optimisation, which I would utilise aggressively. For early cancers without neoadjuvant indication, I would balance the modest delay (4-6 weeks smoking cessation, diabetes optimisation) against progression risk. I would not infer a specific benefit from these observational leak rates; the decision to delay would rest on stage, treatment pathway, physiological status and multidisciplinary discussion."

Q: "How would you counsel a patient who refuses to quit smoking?"
A: "I would counsel the patient that the major risk we worry about in a smoker having this operation is pulmonary — pneumonia, a prolonged period on the ventilator, and respiratory failure. The anastomotic leak rate is also significantly higher; in this cohort it was 15% for smokers versus 5% for non-smokers. I would explain that both types of complication can mean an ICU stay, delayed recovery, the possibility of further surgery, and a risk of death. I would offer smoking cessation support with nicotine replacement and counselling, and explain that stopping smoking for at least four weeks before surgery is one of the most effective things they can do to lower their risk of these complications. If they still decline and the cancer is operable, I would not refuse surgery. I would instead optimise their perioperative respiratory care, have a lower threshold for a feeding jejunostomy or nasojejunal tube in patients at higher nutritional risk, and have a clear plan for managing complications: initial resuscitation and source control, then investigation with contrast swallow or CT, drainage where appropriate, endoscopic management for a contained leak, and takedown with diversion if there is conduit necrosis or uncontrolled sepsis."

Q: "Could confounding explain these associations?"
A: "Absolutely — this is a critical limitation. Smoking correlates with poor nutrition, alcohol use, and COPD. Obesity correlates with OSA and cardiac disease. Poor diabetes control suggests compliance issues. Ideally, I'd want to see multivariable regression adjusting for age, ASA, neoadjuvant therapy, and comorbidities to identify independent predictors. The dose-response relationship across all three factors does suggest genuine causal relationships, but definitive proof would require randomised trials of preoperative optimisation — which would be challenging ethically and practically."

KEY LEARNING POINTS

- ✓ Grouped bar charts show **trends across categories**
- ✓ Always calculate **ARR + RRR**, not just look at p-values

- ✓ Dose-response relationships strengthen **causality arguments**
- ✓ Several modifiable factors matter, but marginal rates **cannot simply be summed**
- ✓ Observational data = **correlation not causation**

BREAST SURGERY

Example 2: Scatter Plot — Oncotype DX Score vs Chemotherapy Benefit

Clinical Scenario:

Illustrative scatter plot demonstrating the conceptual relationship between a genomic recurrence score and modelled chemotherapy benefit in early-stage breast cancer. This is a constructed teaching example and does not represent data from any specific trial. The three-zone interpretation (low / intermediate / high risk) reflects how genomic tools are used in practice. Note that the randomised evidence for Oncotype DX supports identifying patients who can safely omit chemotherapy rather than quantifying how much benefit chemotherapy confers.

Chemotherapy Benefit vs Oncotype DX Score

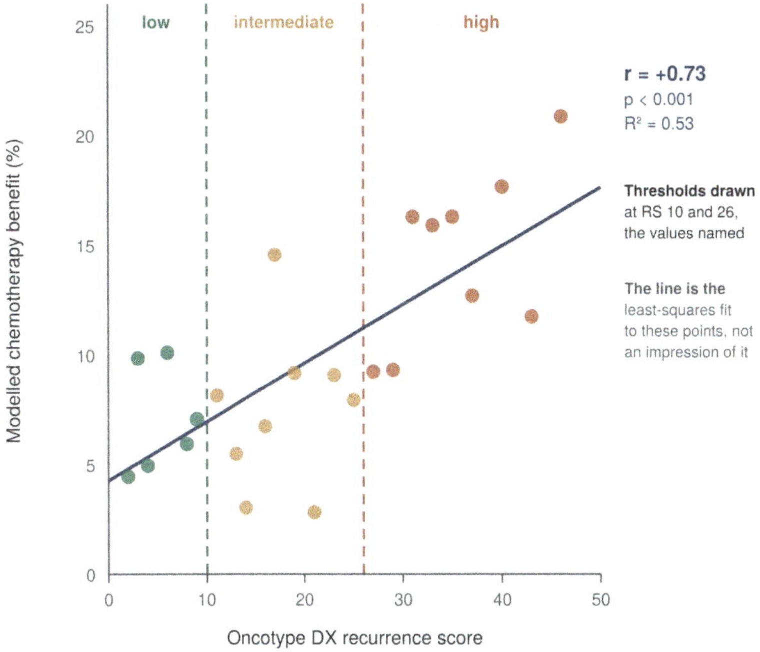

Constructed teaching example, not trial data · TAILORx randomised only the intermediate band, so no randomised estimate of chemotherapy benefit exists above RS 26: that evidence rests on a retrospective NSABP B-20 subgroup, and varies with age and nodal status.

5-SECOND RECOGNITION DRILL

What you see: Dots trending upward from left to right with vertical threshold lines

What it means: As Oncotype score increases → chemotherapy benefit increases

Key pattern: Three distinct zones (low, intermediate and high risk)

Viva opener: "This scatter plot illustrates the relationship between a genomic recurrence score and chemotherapy benefit. In practice, higher Oncotype DX scores are associated with greater absolute benefit from adjuvant chemotherapy, though the randomised evidence is strongest for identifying who can safely omit it"

PERFECT 60-SECOND MODEL VIVA RESPONSE

"This scatter plot is a constructed teaching example illustrating the relationship between a genomic recurrence score and absolute chemotherapy benefit. In clinical practice, higher recurrence scores are associated with greater absolute benefit from adjuvant chemotherapy. The relationship shown here is drawn for teaching purposes and is not trial data.

Three zones are evident:

1. Low risk (RS 0-10): Chemotherapy can be safely omitted. These patients were not randomised in TAILORx; all received endocrine therapy alone, with excellent outcomes.
2. Intermediate (RS 11-25): This is the only band randomised in TAILORx. Endocrine therapy alone was non-inferior overall, with age a major effect modifier — no benefit above 50, a modest one below among women with recurrence scores of 16 to 25.
3. High risk (RS ≥26): Chemotherapy is recommended, but these patients were assigned to it rather than randomised. They form an observational cohort within TAILORx, not a randomised comparison, so the trial cannot estimate the benefit of giving it.

Interpretation depends on the patient, not the score alone. Age and menopausal status govern how the randomised evidence applies: in the intermediate band the benefit of chemotherapy differs above and below 50, and in node-positive disease menopausal status is the dominant modifier. Nodal status, clinical risk, fitness, comorbidity and patient preference all sit alongside the genomic score in the decision.

The point worth making about a patient with a high score is a structural one. TAILORx randomised only the intermediate band, so there is no randomised estimate of chemotherapy benefit at RS 35; the evidence for the high-risk group rests on a retrospective subgroup of NSABP B-20. I would therefore recommend chemotherapy but be honest that the size of the benefit is less precisely established than the low-risk evidence for omitting it — and I would weigh it against age, fitness, comorbidities and preference.

What the assay does and does not tell you. The 21-gene assay measures expression of genes involved in proliferation, ER signalling, HER2 and invasion. It gives a prognostic estimate of distant recurrence risk. In the low- and intermediate-risk groups it helps identify patients for whom that risk is low enough that chemotherapy can be safely omitted. It does not give a randomised, precise estimate of chemotherapy benefit at any given score — least of all above RS 26, where the evidence is retrospective — and it does not replace clinical judgement.

The scatter pattern also shows individual variation — some high-risk patients derive minimal benefit (points below the line), suggesting additional unmeasured factors. This reminds us that genomic testing informs but doesn't dictate — we must integrate with clinical judgement."

⚠ CRITICAL EXAMINER TRAPS

TRAP #1: "Correlation = Causation"

✗ WRONG: ~~"High Oncotype scores CAUSE better chemotherapy response"~~

✓ RIGHT: "High Oncotype scores are prognostic for recurrence risk, and help identify who can safely omit chemotherapy. The score reflects tumour biology — proliferation, ER signalling, HER2 — which determines chemosensitivity. The score doesn't cause response; it identifies biology associated with response."

TRAP #2: "Apply rigidly to all patients"

✗ **WRONG:** ~~"All patients with RS<26 should avoid chemotherapy"~~

✓ **RIGHT:** "Oncotype is one tool among many. For a 35-year-old with RS=24, I might still recommend chemotherapy given her young age and years at risk. For a 75-year-old with RS=28 and significant comorbidities, I might discuss omitting chemotherapy despite high-risk score. The test informs, doesn't mandate."

TRAP #3: Ignoring confidence in estimates

✗ **WRONG:** ~~"RS=25 means exactly 10% benefit"~~

✓ RIGHT: "Any estimate of benefit at a given score carries uncertainty, and in the intermediate band it varies with age. That is why scores of 11-25 require individualised discussion rather than an algorithmic decision."

PERFECT 60-SECOND SUMMARY FOR EXAM

"This scatter plot illustrates the relationship between recurrence score and chemotherapy benefit; it is constructed for teaching and is not trial data. Low-risk patients (RS≤10) can omit chemotherapy. The intermediate zone (11-25) is the only band randomised in TAILORx, where endocrine therapy alone proved non-inferior and age is a major effect modifier. High-risk patients (RS≥26) are offered chemotherapy, though they were not randomised, so the benefit is less precisely quantified than the evidence for omission. Scatter around the regression line reminds us that genomic testing informs but doesn't dictate — clinical factors and patient preference remain essential."

COLORECTAL SURGERY

Example 3: Pie Chart — Distribution of Colorectal Cancer Presenting Features

Clinical Scenario:

Population-based study of 3,456 newly diagnosed colorectal cancer patients examining mode of presentation. Critical for service planning and screening programme design.

Mode of Presentation in Colorectal Cancer (n=3,456)

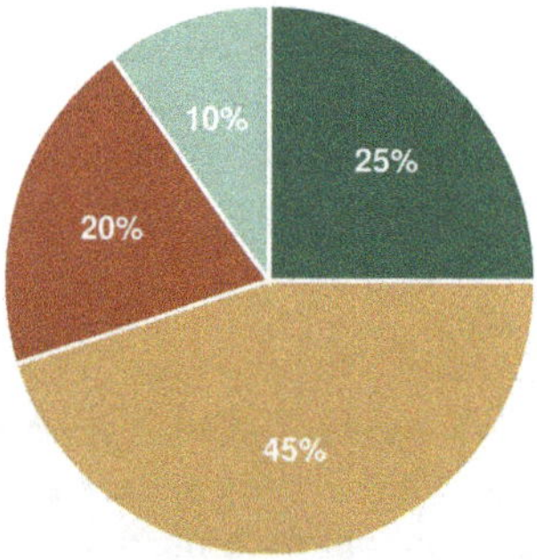

Mode	%	n	Early	5-year
Screening	25%	864	78%	89%
Symptomatic	45%	1,555	52%	64%
Emergency	20%	691	18%	35%
Incidental	10%	346	82%	85%
All	**100%**	**3,456**	**55%**	—

Early = stage I–II at diagnosis

One in five present as an emergency — 691 patients

n = 3,456 · the survival column cannot be compared across rows. Screening advances the diagnosis date (lead-time bias), preferentially finds slow-growing tumours (length-time bias), and detects some cancers that would never have caused harm (overdiagnosis). Whether screening saves lives is answered by mortality in randomised trials, not by these figures.

Chart E3. Mode of presentation in 3,456 patients with colorectal cancer, with stage and survival alongside. The pie shows only the marginal proportions; the value is in the table. Survival falls from 89% in screen-detected to 35% in emergency presentations, but that gradient cannot be read as the benefit of screening — lead-time bias, length-time bias and overdiagnosis all inflate survival among screen-detected cancers, and aggressive tumours arising between screening rounds surface as emergencies. Illustrative data · a constructed teaching example, not a real study.

5-SECOND RECOGNITION DRILL

What you see: Circle divided into coloured slices with percentages
What it means: Proportions of a whole — how patients present
Key pattern: Nearly half present symptomatically, one-quarter screening-detected
Red flag: 20% emergency presentations — missed opportunities
Viva opener: "This pie chart reveals that only 25% of colorectal cancers are screen-detected, with 20% presenting as emergencies — highlighting the ongoing need to improve screening uptake"

PERFECT 60-SECOND MODEL VIVA RESPONSE

"This pie chart from 3,456 colorectal cancer patients reveals critical service planning insights. The distribution shows:

- **25% screen-detected:** Despite national screening programmes, only one-quarter are caught through screening. However, these patients have excellent outcomes — 78% present with Stage I-II disease and 89% 5-year survival. — but see the biases below before treating that as the effect of screening.
- **45% symptomatic:** Nearly half present with symptoms prompting investigation. Stage distribution (52% early) and survival (64%) are intermediate.
- **20% emergency:** This is the most concerning slice. One in five patients present acutely with obstruction, perforation, or bleeding. Only 18% have early-stage disease, and five-year survival is just 35%; 30-day mortality among those undergoing emergency surgery is around 15%. Some of these are missed opportunities, but many are aggressive interval cancers that arose between screening rounds, or patients outside the screening age range — they are not all screening failures
- **10% incidental:** Found during investigations for other conditions. Excellent stage distribution (82% early) and outcomes similar to screening.

The tempting conclusion — that converting emergency presentations to screen-detected would lift survival from 35% to 89% — is a TRAP, and naming it is what scores here. Comparing five-year survival across detection modes is confounded by lead-time bias (screening advances the diagnosis date, so survival is measured from earlier and looks longer even if death occurs at the same moment), length-time bias (screening preferentially catches slow-growing, better-prognosis tumours, while biologically aggressive cancers surface as emergencies), and overdiagnosis (screening detects some cancers that would never have caused symptoms or death, which inflates survival among screen-detected cases without anyone living a day longer). The survival gap therefore reflects when and which cancers are found, not a treatment effect of screening — so whether screening actually saves lives is a question of mortality reduction in randomised trials, not survival by detection mode. What the data do support, descriptively, is that a fifth of colorectal cancers still present as emergencies with poor stage distribution — a fair argument for improving screening uptake — but the 35%-to-89% figure cannot be read as the size of that benefit. The 20% emergency rate also means our services must maintain acute capacity for complex resections despite screening programmes."

⚠ EXAMINER FOLLOW-UP QUESTIONS

Q: "Why do pie charts get criticised in scientific papers?"

A: "Pie charts are difficult for the human eye to compare slice sizes accurately, especially for similar percentages. Bar charts allow more precise comparison. However, pie charts effectively communicate 'parts of a whole' — here, showing that screening accounts for only one-quarter of presentations. They're useful for high-level proportions but less good for detailed comparisons. For this data, I might prefer a stacked bar chart showing stage distribution within each presentation mode."

Q: "How would you reduce emergency presentations?"

A: "Multi-pronged approach:

1. **Screening uptake:** Target underserved populations, address barriers (access, cultural, fear), improve FIT test completion rates
2. **Symptom awareness:** Public campaigns about red-flag symptoms (blood PR, change in bowel habit, weight loss)
3. **Primary care pathways:** Rapid referral for concerning symptoms, lower threshold for investigation in high-risk groups
4. **Interval cancers:** Review patients who progress between screening cycles — could we screen more frequently in high-risk groups?

Realistically, some emergencies are unavoidable — aggressive tumours, late-onset symptoms, patients outside the screening age range — but reducing the rate further is a reasonable service goal."

Q: "Is the 25% screening detection rate good or bad?"

A: "It's suboptimal, though there is a ceiling. This 25% may reflect:

- Interval cancers (develop between screens)
- Screening failures (cancers missed on colonoscopy)
- Age-related — cancers arising outside the screening age range
- Geographic variation — some areas have poor screening uptake

The last point matters arithmetically: cancers occurring outside the eligible age range can never be screen-detected however good uptake becomes, so screen-detection cannot approach 100%. Some comparable national programmes report higher screen-detected fractions, which suggests room for improvement, but any target should be quoted against current uptake and age-range figures for the programme in question, both of which change."

VASCULAR SURGERY

Example 4: Box Plot — Post-EVAR Quality of Life Scores

Clinical Scenario:

Randomised trial comparing EVAR vs open repair for AAA. Quality of life (QoL) measured using SF-36 physical component score (0-100, higher better) at baseline, 3 months, 12 months, and 24 months post-procedure.

SF-36 Physical Component Score Over Time

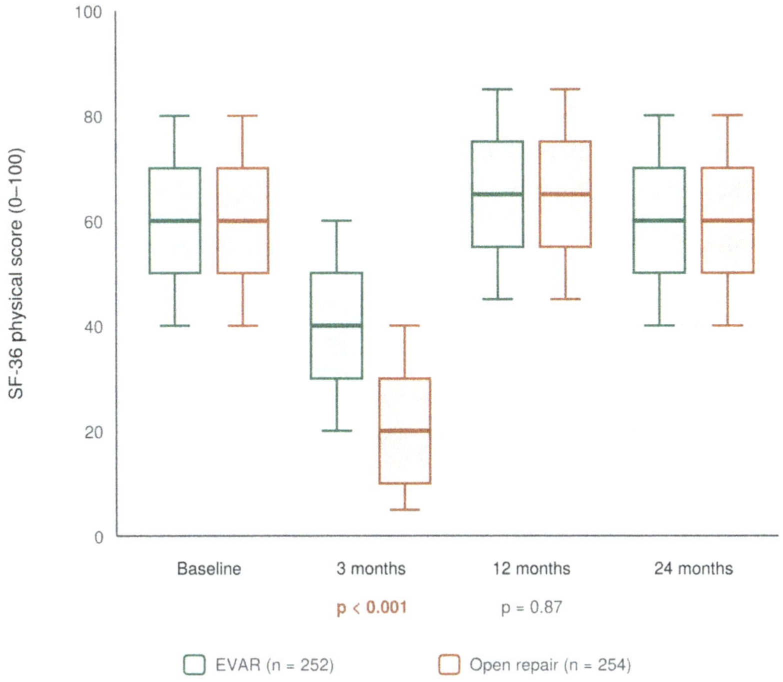

Illustrative data · box = interquartile range, thick line = median, whiskers = range of non-outlying values. Every box carries both whiskers.

How to read box plots: Box = middle 50% (IQR), thick line = median, whiskers = non-outlying range (commonly 1.5×IQR), dots = outliers

5-SECOND RECOGNITION DRILL

What you see: Boxes with whiskers, EVAR (left box) vs Open (right box) at four time points

What it means: Distribution of quality of life scores over time

Key pattern: Open repair dips dramatically at 3 months, then recovers; EVAR shows less decline

Viva opener: "This box plot demonstrates the short-term quality of life advantage of EVAR, with convergence by 12 months"

PERFECT 60-SECOND MODEL VIVA RESPONSE

"This box plot compares quality of life trajectories following EVAR versus open AAA repair over 24 months. Several key patterns emerge:

Baseline: Both groups start similarly — median SF-36 score 60, IQR 50-70. That is reassuring, but baseline balance is not proof that randomisation worked.

3 months: Dramatic divergence. Open repair patients experience substantial QoL decline — median drops to 20 with an IQR of 10-30. EVAR patients fare much better with median 40, IQR 30-50. The difference is unlikely to be chance ($p<0.001$). This reflects the larger incision, longer recovery, and higher complication burden of open repair.

12 months: Convergence. Both groups have not merely recovered but sit slightly above their own baseline, median 65 with an IQR of 55-75 in each arm. The difference is no longer statistically significant ($p=0.87$). This is the critical timepoint — the short-term EVAR advantage disappears.

24 months: Both groups have returned to baseline function, median 60 and IQR 50-70 in each arm. No difference in long-term quality of life was detected, which is not the same as demonstrating equivalence — the trial was not designed to show it.

Clinical interpretation: EVAR offers a clear quality of life advantage at three months that has disappeared by twelve; the trial measured at three, twelve and twenty-four months, so the crossover point between them is not observed. For a 75-year-old with limited life expectancy, that early recovery matters enormously. For a 65-year-old with 15+ years life expectancy, the equivalent long-term outcomes combined with EVAR's higher reintervention rates might favour open repair if anatomically suitable."

⚠ KEY VIVA POINTS ABOUT BOX PLOTS

1. Understanding the Components

- **Bottom whisker:** lowest non-outlying value (commonly 1.5×IQR below Q1, the Tukey convention)
- **Bottom of box:** 25th percentile (Q1)
- **Thick line in box:** Median (50th percentile) — NOT mean!
- **Top of box:** 75th percentile (Q3)
- **Box height (IQR):** Spread of middle 50% of data

- **Top whisker:** highest non-outlying value (commonly 1.5×IQR above Q3, the Tukey convention)
- **Dots beyond whiskers:** Outliers

2. What Box Width/Height Means

- **Tall box:** High variability in middle 50% of patients
- **Short box:** Patients similar to each other
- **Long whiskers:** Wide overall range
- **Asymmetric box:** Skewed distribution

3. Examiner Follow-Up: "Why use box plots instead of bar charts?"

Answer: "Bar charts with error bars only show mean±SD, hiding the distribution shape. Box plots reveal:

- The median (more robust to outliers than mean)
- The spread (IQR shows where middle half of patients lie)
- Skewness (asymmetric boxes indicate non-normal distribution)
- Outliers (individual extreme values visible)

For QoL data, which is often skewed, box plots are superior to simple bar charts."

INSTANT INTERPRETATION FRAMEWORK

1. **Compare medians** (thick lines) — is one group consistently higher/lower?
2. **Check overlap — do the boxes overlap or separate? Overlap is descriptive only; it is not a test of significance**
3. **Assess variability** — is one group more variable (taller boxes)?
4. **Note outliers** — are there extreme individuals?
5. **Track over time** — do groups converge or diverge?

Example 5: ROC Curve — Predicting Symptomatic Carotid Stenosis

Clinical Scenario:

Development of clinical prediction model for symptomatic carotid stenosis requiring intervention. Model uses age, stenosis degree, plaque morphology, and microemboli on TCD. ROC curve assesses discrimination ability.

ROC Curve: Prediction Model for Symptomatic Carotid Events

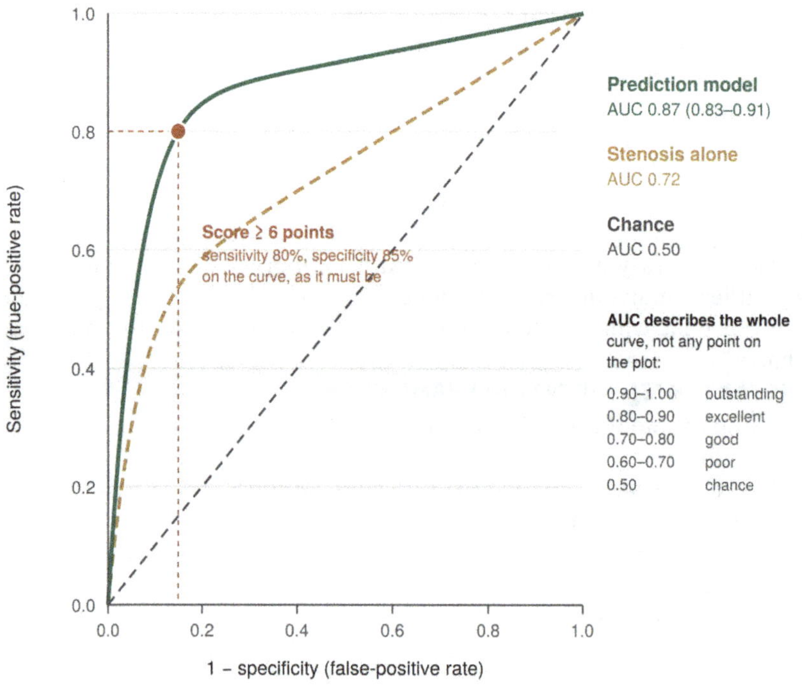

Illustrative data · both curves lie above the chance diagonal, as any test better than guessing must. The marked threshold lies on the curve, because the curve is the set of all thresholds of the same marker. Area measures ranking, not calibration.

UNDERSTANDING ROC CURVES — QUICK GUIDE

AUC Value	Discrimination	Clinical Interpretation
0.90-1.0	Outstanding	Extremely strong discrimination — a powerful decision aid, but still requires external validation and clinical context; it does not replace clinical judgement.
0.80-0.90	Excellent	Model highly useful — strong tool for decision-making
0.70-0.80	Good	Model acceptable — useful adjunct to clinical judgement
0.60-0.70	Poor	Model weak — limited clinical utility
0.50-0.60	No	Barely better than chance

AUC Value	Discrimination	Clinical Interpretation
	discrimination	

5-SECOND RECOGNITION DRILL

What you see: Curved line bowing toward top-left corner with diagonal reference line

What it means: Trade-off between sensitivity (catching all cases) and specificity (avoiding false alarms)

Key pattern: the further the curve sits above the diagonal, the better the discrimination; a curve on the diagonal discriminates no better than chance

Instant assessment: AUC >0.8 means good discrimination. Whether the test is clinically useful is a separate question, and depends on prevalence, the cost of each error and whether the result changes management

Viva opener: "This ROC curve demonstrates excellent discrimination with AUC 0.87, indicating the prediction model reliably identifies high-risk patients"

PERFECT 60-SECOND MODEL VIVA RESPONSE

"This ROC curve evaluates a clinical prediction model for symptomatic carotid stenosis. The model incorporates age, stenosis severity, plaque morphology, and TCD microemboli to generate a risk score.

The AUC of 0.87 (95% CI: 0.83-0.91) indicates excellent discrimination. This means if I randomly select one patient who develops symptoms and one who doesn't, the model will correctly assign a higher risk score to the symptomatic patient 87% of the time. This is significantly better than the stenosis-alone model (AUC 0.72, the lower curve), demonstrating added value of the comprehensive assessment.

The optimal operating point, marked on the curve, occurs at a threshold score of 6 points, yielding 80% sensitivity and 85% specificity. This means:

- Sensitivity 80%: We correctly identify 4 out of 5 patients who will develop symptoms
- Specificity 85%: We correctly reassure 17 out of 20 patients who won't develop symptoms

In this illustrative model, a threshold of ≥6 identifies a higher-risk group who might be considered for expedited assessment alongside intensive medical therapy, while those below it could be managed with optimal medical therapy and surveillance. I would stress that this is a constructed teaching example rather than a validated rule: the threshold itself would need external validation and an assessment of clinical utility before it guided any management decision.

Important caveat: this needs external validation. Discrimination often falls when a model meets a new population, through overfitting, different case mix and changed predictor–outcome relationships. I'd want to see validation in an independent cohort before widespread implementation."

⚠ CRITICAL EXAMINER QUESTIONS & ANSWERS

Q1: "How do you choose the optimal threshold?"

A: "It depends on clinical context and consequences of errors:

- **Cancer screening:** Prioritise sensitivity — can't miss cancers even if more false positives (anxiety, biopsies)
- **Confirmatory test before surgery:** Prioritise specificity — don't want unnecessary operations
- **Carotid stenosis:** Balance is reasonable — high sensitivity catches most at-risk patients; high specificity avoids unnecessary intervention in low-risk patients.

The optimal point mathematically is often where Youden index (Sensitivity + Specificity − 1) is maximised. Here at 80% + 85% − 1 = 0.65. But clinical judgement may favour shifting threshold based on risk tolerance."

Q2: "What's the difference between AUC and accuracy?"

A: "Crucial distinction:

- **Accuracy:** (TP + TN) / Total — percentage correctly classified. Misleading if outcomes unbalanced (e.g., 5% event rate — predicting 'no event' for everyone gives 95% accuracy but useless clinically)
- **AUC:** Threshold-independent — assesses discrimination across ALL possible thresholds. Much more robust measure of model performance

AUC also has intuitive interpretation — probability model correctly ranks a random case-control pair. But discrimination is only half the story: AUC should be read alongside calibration and clinical usefulness, since a model can rank patients well and still give badly miscalibrated risks."

Q3: "The CI is 0.83-0.91. What if it was 0.70-0.95?"

A: "Wide CI indicates imprecision — small sample size or high variability. While point estimate looks good (AUC 0.87), true performance could be merely 'acceptable' (0.70) or outstanding (0.95). This uncertainty undermines confidence in the model. I would want larger validation sample to narrow the CI before implementing clinically. Narrow CI (0.83-0.91) in our example gives confidence the model truly performs in the 'excellent' range."

Q4: "How would you validate this model?"

A: "Multi-step process:

1. **Internal validation:** Bootstrap or cross-validation in derivation cohort — corrects for optimism
2. **Temporal validation:** Test on more recent patients from same centre — ensures model hasn't drifted

3. **External validation:** Apply to different centre/population — tests generalisability
4. **Calibration:** Not just discrimination (AUC) but also calibration — do predicted risks match observed risks? Plot calibration curve
5. **Clinical impact:** Decision curve analysis — does model improve decisions vs. treat-all or treat-none strategies?
Only after robust validation would I recommend implementation in clinical pathways."

KEY LEARNING POINTS — ROC CURVES

- ✓ **AUC interpretation:** Probability of correctly ranking a random case-control pair
- ✓ **Diagonal line (AUC=0.5):** No discrimination — random guessing
- ✓ **Perfect test (AUC=1.0):** Curve goes to top-left corner
- ✓ **Threshold choice:** Clinical context determines optimal sensitivity/specificity balance
- ✓ **Model comparison:** Can plot multiple ROC curves to compare models
- ✓ **Confidence intervals:** Wide CI = imprecise estimate, need larger sample
- ✓ **External validation:** Essential before clinical implementation

ROC CURVE INSTANT INTERPRETATION CHECKLIST

1. Check AUC: below 0.70 is poor discrimination; 0.70–0.79 is good; 0.80 and above is excellent. These describe discrimination only — there is no AUC at which a test becomes clinically useful, because that depends on prevalence, the cost of each error, calibration and whether the result changes management
2. **Assess CI width:** Narrow = precise, wide = uncertain
3. **Locate optimal point:** Where would you set threshold clinically?
4. **Compare to alternatives:** Better than existing tests/models?
5. **Consider validation:** Internal only or externally validated?

HPB SURGERY

Example 6: Funnel Plot — Publication Bias in Liver Resection Meta-Analysis

Clinical Scenario:

Meta-analysis of 28 studies comparing laparoscopic vs open liver resection for colorectal metastases. Outcomes reported: overall survival, perioperative mortality, and hospital stay. Funnel plot assesses publication bias.

Funnel Plot: Overall Survival — Laparoscopic vs Open Liver Resection

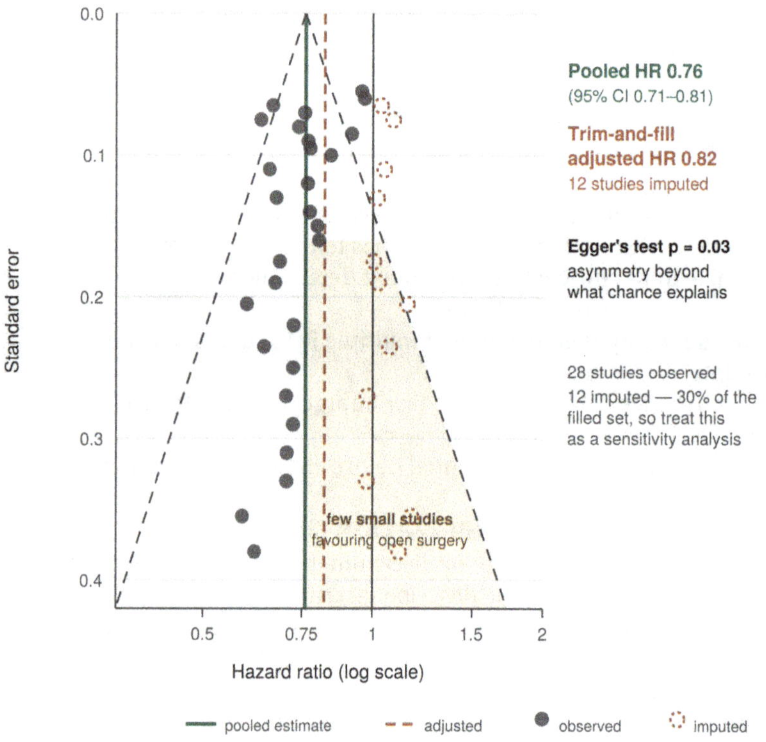

Illustrative data · random-effects pooling. Trim-and-fill imputes studies under its own assumptions; it does not establish that any are missing. Asymmetry can also arise from heterogeneity or poorer methods in small trials, not only from publication bias.

⚠ WHAT THIS ASYMMETRY MEANS

The gap in the bottom-right corner indicates small studies showing laparoscopic is WORSE (or no benefit) are missing from the published literature. If that gap reflects suppression, it would mean the apparent benefit is inflated from HR=0.82 (adjusted) to HR=0.76 (observed) — but asymmetry alone does not establish the cause. While benefit persists after adjustment, it's smaller than initially appears.

5-SECOND RECOGNITION DRILL

What you see: Inverted funnel/triangle with dots scattered inside, gap on one side at bottom

What it means: Testing whether small negative studies are missing (publication bias)
Key pattern: a gap at the bottom on one side is asymmetry. Publication bias is one explanation; heterogeneity, poorer methods in small trials and chance are others. Symmetry does not exclude bias either
Red flag: Missing small studies on right (favouring control) suggests selective publishing
Viva opener: "This funnel plot shows asymmetry, with Egger's test p=0.03. Publication bias is one possible cause, and if it is the cause the benefit is overestimated"

PERFECT 60-SECOND MODEL VIVA RESPONSE

"This funnel plot evaluates publication bias in a meta-analysis of laparoscopic versus open liver resection. Each dot represents one study, plotted by effect size (x-axis) and precision/sample size (y-axis).
In the absence of bias, we expect symmetric distribution around the pooled estimate — a funnel shape with large studies clustered at the top (high precision) and small studies scattered widely at the bottom (low precision).
However, this plot shows clear asymmetry. The most precise studies scatter around the pooled estimate. But small studies at the bottom are predominantly on the LEFT side (favouring laparoscopic), with a conspicuous gap on the RIGHT (favouring open or showing no benefit).
This pattern is consistent with publication bias — small negative studies may exist but remain unpublished because journals and investigators favour positive results. Egger's test at p=0.03 establishes that the asymmetry is unlikely to be chance; it does not establish its cause.
Using trim-and-fill to impute missing studies (shown as open circles), the adjusted estimate becomes HR=0.82 versus the observed HR=0.76 — approximately 18% versus 24% reduction in hazard. But that requires imputing twelve studies onto twenty-eight observed, so almost a third of the filled dataset is invented. Treat it as a sensitivity analysis, not a corrected result.
Clinically, I would still recommend laparoscopic approach for suitable patients, as even the conservative adjusted estimate shows significant benefit. However, I would counsel patients that published literature may overstate the advantage, with the adjusted estimate sitting closer to the null, because of selective publication. This underscores the importance of trial registration and mandated reporting of negative results."

⚠ CRITICAL EXAMINER QUESTIONS — PUBLICATION BIAS

Q1: "What CAUSES publication bias?"
A: "Multiple mechanisms:

1. **File-drawer effect:** Investigators don't submit negative studies, assuming journals won't accept them
2. **Journal bias:** Editors preferentially accept positive results as more "interesting"
3. **Citation bias:** Positive studies cited more, increasing visibility and impact
4. **Language bias:** Positive studies more likely published in English, negative in local languages
5. **Time-lag bias:** Positive studies published faster than negative
6. **Outcome reporting bias:** Authors selectively report favourable outcomes from multi-outcome trials

The result: published literature can systematically overestimate treatment effects, sometimes substantially, though the magnitude varies between fields and study designs."

Q2: "How can we prevent publication bias?"
A: "Several strategies:

- **Trial registration:** Mandatory pre-registration (ClinicalTrials.gov) commits investigators to publish regardless of results
- **Reporting guidelines:** CONSORT/PRISMA statements require full outcome reporting
- **Results registries:** Require posting of results to registries within 1 year
- **Journal policies:** Journals like PLOS ONE commit to publishing well-conducted negative trials
- **Grey literature search:** Meta-analyses should search conference abstracts, dissertations, trial registries
- **Individual patient data:** Request unpublished IPD directly from investigators"

Q3: "Are there other explanations for funnel plot asymmetry besides publication bias?"
A: "Yes — important differential diagnosis:

- **Heterogeneity:** Small studies in different populations/settings with genuinely different effects
- **Poor methodological quality:** Small studies often have weaker methods, inflating effects
- **Chance:** Random scatter, especially with <10 studies (Cochrane guidance)
- **True effect modification:** Small studies conducted in higher-risk populations where treatment effects are genuinely larger — asymmetry here reflects real biology, not missing trials."

MODULE 2: Advanced Statistical Concepts

Quick reference cards covering proportional hazards assumptions, non-inferiority trials, intention-to-treat analysis, multiple comparisons, survival analysis, publication bias, and Bayesian vs Frequentist statistics. Each card includes viva phrases and examiner TRAPs.

Card 1: The Proportional Hazards Assumption

In Plain English:
"If treatment reduces your risk of death by 25% at 1 year, it should reduce it by 25% at 5 years too."

⚠ When It's Violated

- **Crossing curves:** Kaplan–Meier curves cross over time
- **Early harm, late benefit:** Surgery complications early, survival benefit late
- **Delayed effect:** Immunotherapy takes months to work
- **Waning benefit:** Treatment effect diminishes over time

How to Test It

Method	What It Does
Schoenfeld residuals test	Statistical test ($p<0.05$ counts against proportionality; $p \geq 0.05$ is not proof of it)
Log-log plot	Lines should be parallel
Visual inspection	Check if KM curves cross

VIVA PHRASE:
"The proportional hazards assumption requires that the hazard ratio remains constant over follow-up. The Schoenfeld test p-value of 0.003 indicates violation, suggesting time-varying effects (illustrative violation example — a significant p-value here means the assumption is not met). I would examine a time-varying hazard ratio plot to understand when the treatment effect changes."

✗ EXAMINER TRAP:
Don't just say "proportional hazards violated" without explaining what it means clinically. Always interpret: "This suggests treatment benefit emerges gradually" or "Early harm from surgery is offset by late survival benefit."

What to Do If Violated

1. **Time-varying Cox model:** Allow HR to change over time
2. **Restricted mean survival time:** Alternative to HR
3. **Landmark analysis:** Analyse from specific timepoint
4. **Stratified Cox:** Separate models for early/late periods

> **Viva phrase**: "If proportional hazards is violated, a single hazard ratio may obscure important changes in the treatment effect over time. I would want to see how that effect varies during follow-up, and I would consider a time-varying treatment effect or another approach suited to non-proportional hazards."

Card 2: Non-Inferiority vs Superiority Trials

The Key Difference

Trial Type	Hypothesis	Example
Superiority	New treatment is BETTER	Chemo + surgery > surgery alone
Non-Inferiority	New treatment is NOT WORSE by more than a margin	Laparoscopic not worse than open (within 5%)
Equivalence	Two treatments have SIMILAR effects	Generic drug = brand name

Why Non-Inferiority?
Used when new treatment offers **other advantages**:
- Less invasive (laparoscopic vs open)
- Fewer side effects
- Lower cost
- Easier administration

We accept slightly lower efficacy IF not clinically meaningful.

The Non-Inferiority Margin

Δ = Maximum acceptable difference

> **⚠ The question examiners actually ask: how was the margin justified?**

The margin *is* the appraisal. Set it generously and a clearly worse treatment passes as "non-inferior." A defensible margin is justified in the protocol on four grounds:

- **Preservation of effect** — it preserves a clinically important proportion of the standard treatment's established benefit over placebo or no treatment, judged against reliable historical evidence.

There is no universal percentage: a margin justified by an arbitrary fraction rather than by the evidence is one an examiner can challenge.

- **Clinical meaningfulness** — the loss it tolerates is one clinicians and patients would genuinely accept in exchange for the new treatment's advantages (less invasive, cheaper, better tolerated).

- **Pre-specified** — fixed before unblinding, never chosen to fit the result.
- **Assay sensitivity and constancy** — the trial must be capable of telling an effective treatment from an ineffective one, and the standard treatment must perform broadly as the historical evidence predicts. If the control arm does unexpectedly badly, the two treatments can look similar simply because neither worked, and apparent non-inferiority becomes meaningless.

Note also that **intention-to-treat can *flatter* non-inferiority**: dropouts and crossovers blur the groups towards each other, pushing the result towards "no difference." Per-protocol analysis has the opposite problem: it breaks randomisation. Neither is safe alone, which is why a non-inferiority claim should hold in both, and concordant conclusions from the two analyses are what give it credibility (see Card 3).

Viva phrase: "My first question in any non-inferiority trial is how the margin was justified. I would want to know whether it preserves a clinically important proportion of the standard treatment's established effect, whether the loss it tolerates is one patients would genuinely accept in exchange for the new treatment's advantages, whether it was pre-specified, and whether assay sensitivity was maintained — that the control arm performed as the historical evidence predicts. I would then look for concordant intention-to-treat and per-protocol analyses. A margin that tolerates a clinically unacceptable loss makes the conclusion meaningless, however tight the confidence interval."

Example: Δ = 5% for mortality

If new treatment mortality is 15% and standard is 10%, difference is 5% — just at the margin.

Interpreting CI in Non-Inferiority

Scenario: Non-inferiority margin = +5%

Result: Difference = -2% (95% CI: -4% to +1%)

- ✓ **Upper CI (+1%) is within margin (+5%)** → Non-inferiority proven
- ⚠ CI crosses zero → not superior, just non-inferior

In this example the outcome is a complication rate (higher value = worse), so the upper CI bound is decisive — it must stay within the inferiority margin.

If CI was (-1% to +7%):

- ✗ Upper CI (+7%) exceeds margin (+5%) → Non-inferiority NOT proven — we cannot exclude that the new treatment causes 7% more complications, which is beyond the acceptable margin.
- *Note: in both scenarios on this card, the outcome is a complication rate (higher=worse), so the* ***upper*** *CI bound is decisive — it must stay within the margin. For outcomes where lower=worse (e.g. survival, cure, or response rate), the* ***lower*** *CI bound is decisive instead. Match the bound to the direction of harm.*

PERFECT VIVA ANSWER:
"This is a non-inferiority trial with a pre-specified margin of 5%. The 95% confidence interval upper bound is 1%, which lies within the +5% margin, confirming non-inferiority. Laparoscopic surgery was not shown to be superior; what the trial supports is that it is not worse by more than the pre-specified margin, alongside reduced pain, shorter stay, and faster recovery — making it the preferred approach."

✗ COMMON ERROR:
Don't interpret non-inferiority as "treatments are equal" — it means "new treatment not unacceptably worse." Big difference!

⚠ Critical Issue: Assay Sensitivity

Non-inferiority requires that the **control arm performs as expected** from historical data. If control arm does unexpectedly well/poorly, the trial loses assay sensitivity.
Example TRAP: If standard treatment usually gives 80% survival but in this trial gives 90%, then "proving non-inferiority" is easier but meaningless!

Card 3: ITT vs Per-Protocol Analysis

The Fundamental Principle

Intention-to-Treat (ITT):
Analyse patients in the groups they were randomised to, regardless of what actually happened.
Per-Protocol (PP): Analyse only patients who **completed treatment as planned**.

Example Scenario

100 patients randomised to laparoscopic surgery:
- 15 converted to open
- 5 refused surgery
- 2 died before surgery

- 78 completed laparoscopic surgery

Analysis Type	N analysed in Lap group	Effect
ITT	100 (all randomised)	Conservative, realistic
PP	78 (completed only)	Optimistic, ideal scenario

✓ Advantages of ITT

- **Preserves randomisation** — groups remain comparable
- **Reflects real-world** — includes all treatment failures
- **Prevents bias** — can't cherry-pick successful patients
- **Preferred primary analysis for most superiority trials**

⚠ Disadvantages of ITT

- **Dilutes effect:** Includes patients who never got treatment
- **Bias toward null:** May miss real treatment effects
- **Unfair if many crossovers:** Mixes intervention with control

When Each is Appropriate

Use ITT for:

- ✓ Superiority trials
- ✓ Pragmatic trials (real-world effectiveness)
- ✓ When treatment compliance varies

Use Per-Protocol for:

- ⚠ Non-inferiority trials (as sensitivity analysis)
- ⚠ Efficacy trials (does it work under ideal conditions?)
- ⚠ When ITT would be misleading (massive crossover)

VIVA RESPONSE:
"This trial used intention-to-treat analysis, which is appropriate for a superiority trial. All 503 randomised patients are included regardless of treatment completion. While 146 of the 250 patients in the chemotherapy arm didn't complete all six cycles, including them reflects real-world practice where some patients can't tolerate full treatment. This gives us an honest estimate of effectiveness if we offer chemotherapy, knowing some will discontinue."

⚠ CRITICAL FOR NON-INFERIORITY:
In a non-inferiority trial, ITT biases results towards no difference and so favours a conclusion of non-inferiority. Must analyse BOTH ITT and PP — non-inferiority must hold in both to be convincing.

Modified ITT (mITT)

Compromise approach: Exclude patients who never received ANY treatment (e.g., found inoperable at laparotomy) but include all others.

Examiner question: "Is mITT acceptable?"
Answer: "Depends on reason for exclusion. Excluding patients found to have metastases at laparotomy is reasonable — they were ineligible from start. But excluding patients who refused treatment or had complications is not — these are treatment failures that should count."

Card 4: Multiple Testing Problem & Corrections

The Problem: If you test 20 hypotheses at p=0.05, you expect 1 "significant" result by chance alone!

This is why subgroup analyses and fishing expeditions are dangerous.

The Maths: Probability of ≥1 false positive = $1 - (0.95)^n$ where n = number of tests

Number of Tests	Chance of ≥1 False Positive
1	5%
5	23%
10	40%
20	64%
100	99.4%

Correction Methods

1. Bonferroni Correction

Adjusted $\alpha = 0.05 / n$
Example: 10 tests → require $p < 0.005$

- ✓ Simple, conservative
- ✗ Very conservative (loses power)
- ✗ Conservative when tests are correlated (it is valid under any dependence, but loses power)

2. Holm-Bonferroni (Sequential)

Less conservative than Bonferroni:
1. Order p-values smallest to largest
2. First test: $\alpha = 0.05/n$
3. Second test: $\alpha = 0.05/(n-1)$
4. Continue until test fails, stop there

3. False Discovery Rate (FDR)

Controls proportion of false positives among "significant" results
- Less conservative than Bonferroni

- Good for exploratory analyses
- Commonly used in genomics

When to Apply Corrections

Scenario	Correction Needed?
Pre-specified primary outcome	✗ No
Pre-specified secondary outcomes (3-5)	⚠ Debatable
Multiple subgroup analyses	✓ Yes
Post-hoc exploratory analyses	✓ Yes
Safety outcomes (adverse events)	✗ Usually not

Note on safety outcomes: multiplicity does not disappear because the outcome is a harm. Stringent correction is often inappropriate where the priority is detecting a signal rather than avoiding a false alarm, but the analysis plan should still say in advance how multiple adverse events will be handled.

VIVA ANSWER:

"This study reports 12 subgroup analyses without adjustment for multiple testing. With 12 comparisons at an unadjusted p<0.05 we would expect about 0.6 false positives, and the chance of at least one is 1 – 0.95^12, or roughly 46%. The finding that treatment works in patients under 60 but not over 60 (p=0.04) could be spurious. I would treat this as hypothesis-generating only and require validation in a dedicated trial before changing practice based on age."

⚠ EXAMINER TRAP:

"Should we ALWAYS apply Bonferroni?" NO!

Over-correction loses power and may miss real effects.

Use clinical judgement:

- Pre-specified analyses: often no correction
- Exploratory/subgroups: yes, correct
- Safety monitoring: don't want to miss signals, so less stringent

Smart Alternative: Pre-Specification

Best solution: **Register trial protocol beforehand** stating:

- ONE primary outcome
- 3-5 secondary outcomes (pre-specified)
- Planned subgroups (if any)
- Analysis plan before seeing data

This reduces data dredging and makes the inferential status of each analysis clear. It does not remove multiplicity: twenty pre-specified hypotheses still carry an inflated family-wise error rate.

Card 5: Confounding vs Effect Modification

Two Different Concepts — Don't Confuse!

CONFOUNDING

= Bias

A distortion of the true effect

We want to CONTROL for it

EFFECT MODIFICATION

= Real biology

Treatment works differently in subgroups

We want to IDENTIFY it

CONFOUNDING Explained

Definition:

Variable associated with both exposure AND outcome, creating spurious association.

Classic Example:

- Coffee drinkers have higher lung cancer rates
- Confounded by SMOKING (smokers drink more coffee)
- Smoking is associated with coffee drinking and causes lung cancer, which is what makes it the confounder
- Coffee doesn't cause cancer — association is spurious

Criteria for a Confounder

- Associated with exposure (coffee drinking)
- Associated with outcome (lung cancer)
- NOT on causal pathway (not a mediator)
- Can create or mask true associations

How to Control Confounding

Method	How It Works
Randomisation	Distributes confounders equally (RCTs)
Restriction	Include only non-smokers (limits generalisability)
Matching	Match each coffee drinker to non-drinker of same smoking status
Stratification	Analyse smokers and non-smokers separately
Regression	Multivariable model adjusting for smoking

EFFECT MODIFICATION Explained

Definition:

Treatment effect differs across subgroups defined by a third variable.

Surgical Example:

- Chemotherapy reduces mortality in node-positive patients (HR 0.60)

- But has no effect in node-negative patients (HR 0.95)
- Nodal status MODIFIES the treatment effect
- This is REAL biology, not bias!

How to Detect Effect Modification

Test for INTERACTION
p-interaction < 0.05 = effect modification present
In regression model:
Outcome = Treatment + NodeStatus + (Treatment × NodeStatus)
The interaction term tests if treatment effect differs by node status.

Key Differences Summary

	Confounding	Effect Modification
Nature	Bias/artefact	Real biological phenomenon
Goal	Eliminate it	Identify and report it
Analysis	Adjust/control for	Stratify to show subgroups
Reporting	Report adjusted estimate	Report separate estimates per subgroup
Clinical impact	Correction gives true effect	Guides personalised treatment

VIVA ANSWER — CONFOUNDING:
"Age is a confounder here — older patients are more likely to receive open surgery (exposure) and more likely to have complications (outcome), creating spurious association. The authors appropriately used multivariable regression adjusting for age, and the benefit of laparoscopic surgery persists (OR 0.65), suggesting it's a true effect independent of age."

VIVA ANSWER — EFFECT MODIFICATION:
"The interaction test at p = 0.01 is evidence that nodal status modifies the treatment effect rather than a chance subgroup finding. In a randomised trial that is unlikely to be confounding, though it is still a subgroup result and biological plausibility is an argument, not a proof. Node-positive patients benefit substantially from chemotherapy (HR 0.60). An approximate NNT can be estimated if a baseline event rate is assumed — for example, with a ~50% 5-year mortality in node-positive disease, NNT≈7 (survival 0.50^0.60 = 0.66, so mortality 34% against 50%, an absolute reduction of 16%, giving 6.25 rounded up); but NNT cannot be derived from an HR alone without this assumption, while node-negative patients don't benefit (HR 0.95, NNT>50). This guides practice: I would strongly recommend chemotherapy for node-positive patients but discuss risks and benefits carefully with node-negative patients, where toxicity may outweigh minimal benefit."

Card 6: Survival Analysis — Key Concepts

Why Survival Analysis?

Standard methods can't handle:

- **Censoring:** Not all patients followed to event
- **Time-varying risk:** Risk changes over time
- **Different follow-up:** Patients enter/leave at different times

Key Terms You MUST Know

CENSORING

Patient contributes data for part of study, then "disappears" without event:

- **Right censoring:** Lost to follow-up, withdrew, study ended (most common)
- **Left censoring:** Event occurred before enrolment (rare)
- **Interval censoring:** Event between two visits (unknown exact time)

Key point: Censoring assumes patients censored have same risk as those continuing. If high-risk patients drop out preferentially → bias!

HAZARD VS PROBABILITY

Measure	Meaning	Range
Survival Probability	Chance of surviving to time t	0 to 1 (100%)
Hazard Rate	Instantaneous risk of event at time t (given survival to t)	0 to ∞
Cumulative Hazard	Sum of all hazards up to time t	0 to ∞

Hazard Ratio (HR) Interpretation

HR = Hazard in Treatment / Hazard in Control

HR Value	Interpretation	Example
HR = 1.0	No difference	Equal hazard (no difference in event rate)
HR = 0.75	25% reduction in hazard	Treatment reduces hazard (rate of events)
HR = 0.50	50% reduction in hazard (halves the instantaneous event rate)	Strong benefit
HR = 2.0	Doubles the hazard	Treatment harmful

⚠ CRITICAL:

HR is NOT the same as relative risk!

- HR = rate at which events occur
- RR = proportion who had event by specific time
- When events are rare and follow-up complete, they're similar

- With censoring or competing risks, they differ

Competing Risks — When Kaplan–Meier Overstates

A **competing risk** is an event that *prevents* the outcome you are measuring from ever happening. If you are counting cancer recurrence, a patient who dies of a myocardial infarction can never recur — their recurrence is not merely unobserved, it is impossible.

Standard Kaplan–Meier treats that patient as *censored*, which quietly assumes they could still have recurred later. That assumption inflates the estimated risk of the outcome. The effect is largest exactly where surgeons work: **elderly and comorbid populations**, where death from other causes is common, and in long follow-up.

The correct tool is the **cumulative incidence function (CIF)**, which accounts for competing events; Fine–Gray regression models the subdistribution hazard, which is a related but distinct question from cause-specific hazards. If a paper reports "5-year freedom from recurrence" by Kaplan–Meier in an 80-year-old cohort with substantial non-cancer mortality, the figure is probably optimistic.

VIVA PHRASE

"In this elderly population I would want a competing-risks analysis. If death from another cause prevents the event of interest from ever occurring, it is a competing event rather than ordinary non-informative censoring. Treating it as censoring in a standard Kaplan–Meier analysis can overestimate the cumulative incidence of recurrence, because the method assumes those patients could still have recurred. I would report the cumulative incidence function instead."

Median Survival

Definition: Time at which 50% of patients have experienced event

How to read from Kaplan–Meier curve:

1. Draw horizontal line at 50% survival
2. Where it crosses survival curve, drop vertical line to x-axis
3. That time = median survival

⚠ **Problem:** If survival curve never drops to 50% (e.g., cure), median is "not reached" (NR). Report 5-year or 10-year survival instead.

Log-Rank Test

Statistical test comparing survival curves:

- Tests null hypothesis: curves are identical
- $p < 0.05$ → reject null → curves differ significantly
- Gives OVERALL difference across entire follow-up
- Sensitive to proportional hazards violation (curves crossing)

Cox Proportional Hazards Model

Regression for survival data — allows adjustment for confounders

$h(t) = h_0(t) \times \exp(\beta_1 X_1 + \beta_2 X_2 + \ldots)$

Outputs:

- Hazard ratios for each variable
- Adjusted for other covariates
- Assumes proportional hazards (must check!)

VIVA PHRASE:

"The Cox model gives an adjusted hazard ratio of 0.75 (95% CI: 0.60-0.93), meaning a 25% reduction in hazard of death after adjusting for age, stage, and comorbidities. The Schoenfeld test p=0.45 suggests proportional hazards assumption is met, validating the Cox model (illustrative passing example — a non-significant p-value here means the assumption holds)."

⚠ Common Pitfalls

- ✗ Confusing HR with RR
- ✗ Not checking proportional hazards
- ✗ Interpreting p-value without looking at CI
- ✗ Ignoring informative censoring
- ✗ Comparing medians when curves haven't crossed 50%

Card 7: Publication Bias — Detection & Impact

What Is Publication Bias?

Systematic tendency for studies with positive results to be published, while negative studies remain unpublished.

Result: published literature can overestimate treatment effects, sometimes substantially. The magnitude varies between fields and designs and is not a fixed figure.

Detection Methods

1. Funnel Plot (Visual)

- Plot effect size vs precision
- Should be symmetric funnel
- Asymmetry (gap at bottom) = publication bias
- Cochrane advises at least 10 studies before interpreting asymmetry

Limitation: Asymmetry can also reflect heterogeneity, poor quality in small studies

2. Egger's Test (Statistical)

$p < 0.05$ = significant asymmetry

- Regression-based test
- More objective than visual inspection
- Can give false positives if heterogeneity present

3. Trim-and-Fill Analysis

Imputes "missing" studies to restore symmetry:

- Estimates how many studies missing
- Calculates adjusted pooled estimate
- Compare observed vs adjusted effect

Example: Observed OR=0.65 → Adjusted OR=0.72
— adjustment moves the estimate closer to the null

Prevention Strategies

- **Trial registration:** Pre-register on ClinicalTrials.gov before enrolment
- **Prospective registration:** Protocol uploaded before seeing data
- **Results reporting:** Mandate posting results within 1 year
- **Grey literature search:** Conference abstracts, dissertations, preprints
- **Contact authors:** Request unpublished data directly
- **Journal policies:** PLOS ONE publishes well-conducted negative trials

Impact Assessment

Scenario	Impact	Action
Adjusted effect still significant	Minor bias	Accept findings with caution
Adjusted estimate materially attenuated	Moderate	Use adjusted estimate for counselling
Adjusted CI crosses the null	Major	Question validity
Adjustment rests on a large imputed fraction, or estimators disagree	Severe	Treat as sensitivity analysis only; await definitive evidence

PERFECT VIVA ANSWER:

"The funnel plot shows asymmetry with Egger's test p=0.03, which is consistent with publication bias though other causes exist. Trim-and-fill imputes twelve studies and moves the pooled HR from 0.76 to 0.82, still showing benefit but closer to the null than it first appears. I would treat that adjustment as a sensitivity analysis rather than a corrected result, since almost a third of the filled dataset is imputed, and I would counsel patients on the basis that the published literature may overstate the effect."

⚠ EXAMINER TRAP:

"Does publication bias mean we should reject meta-analysis findings?"
ANSWER:
"Not necessarily. If adjusted effect remains significant and clinically meaningful, findings are still valid — we just temper expectations.

Publication bias is a 'known unknown' we acknowledge and quantify. However, if adjustment eliminates significance entirely, we should question the conclusion and potentially await large definitive trials before changing practice."

Card 8: Bayesian vs Frequentist Interpretation

Fundamental Philosophical Difference

FREQUENTIST

Probability = Long-run frequency

"If we repeated this study infinite times, what proportion would show this result?"

Most clinical trials use this

BAYESIAN

Probability = Degree of belief

"Given this data and prior knowledge, how likely is the hypothesis?"

Emerging in adaptive trials

P-Value Interpretation

Statement	Correct?	Framework
"Probability the null hypothesis is true"	✗	Common error
"Probability of seeing data this extreme IF null true"	✓	Frequentist (correct)
"Probability treatment works given the data"	⚠	Bayesian (need prior)

Key Differences in Practice

FREQUENTIST APPROACH

- **Usually a fixed sample size:** Determine N beforehand, collect all data, analyse once — though group-sequential and adaptive frequentist designs allow prespecified interim analyses
- **P-value:** Probability of data at least as extreme as those observed, if the null hypothesis and the statistical model are true
- **Confidence interval:** If we repeat study 100 times, 95 CIs would contain true value
- **No prior information:** Each trial starts fresh
- **Binary conclusion:** Significant or not (p<0.05 cutoff)

BAYESIAN APPROACH

- **Accumulating data: Bayesian methods update as data arrive and support probability-based decision rules. Adaptive design is a separate concept — adaptive trials may be Bayesian or frequentist**
- **Posterior probability:** Probability hypothesis is true given data
- **Credible interval:** 95% probability true value lies in this range

- **Incorporates prior:** Uses previous studies/knowledge
- **Probability gradient:** "85% probability treatment works"

Bayes' Theorem

P(Hypothesis|Data) = P(Data|Hypothesis) × P(Hypothesis) / P(Data)

In words:

Posterior = Likelihood × Prior / Evidence

Clinical Example

Question: New drug shows p=0.04 in small trial (n=100). How confident should we be?

Frequentist interpretation:

"4% chance of seeing this result if drug doesn't work. Reject null hypothesis."

Bayesian interpretation:

"Depends on prior belief. If prior studies showed no effect (sceptical prior), posterior probability drug works might be only 60%. If biological plausibility high (optimistic prior), might be 85%."

✓ When Bayesian Adds Value

- **Rare diseases:** Can't do large trials, must use prior data
- **Adaptive trials:** Adjust based on accumulating data
- **Futility analysis:** Stop early if low probability of success
- **Personalised medicine:** Incorporate individual patient factors
- **Platform trials:** Multiple arms, shared controls

VIVA ANSWER:

"This trial uses Bayesian adaptive design with interim analyses. The posterior probability of superiority is 94%, meaning given the data and pre-specified sceptical prior, there's 94% probability laparoscopic is better. This is more intuitive than a p-value and allowed early stopping for efficacy at 70% planned enrolment, saving time and resources while maintaining statistical rigour."

⚠ LIMITATIONS OF BAYESIAN:

- Results can depend on the choice of prior, particularly when data are limited, so the prior should be justified and sensitivity to plausible alternatives assessed
- Less familiar to clinicians and regulators
- More complex computationally
- Can be manipulated by biased prior selection

Solution: Pre-specify prior in protocol, use "sceptical" or "non-informative" priors

REFERENCE SECTION A: Study Design Cards

Card 9: Adaptive Trial Designs

What Makes a Trial "Adaptive"?

Allows pre-planned modifications based on accumulating data DURING the trial

Traditional RCT = fixed design, no changes after start
Adaptive RCT = pre-specified rules for modification

Types of Adaptations

1. Sample Size Re-estimation

Problem: Initial power calculation based on assumed effect size. What if actual effect different?

Solution: At interim analysis, re-estimate effect size and adjust final sample size

- ✓ Avoids underpowered trial if effect smaller than expected
- ✓ Can stop early if effect larger than expected
- ⚠ Must control Type I error with alpha spending function

2. Response-Adaptive Randomisation

Concept: Allocate more patients to better-performing arm as data accumulates

Example: Start 1:1 randomisation. If Arm A shows better response, shift to 2:1 favouring Arm A

- ✓ Ethical — fewer patients get inferior treatment
- ✓ Efficient — more information on promising arm
- ✗ Can reduce power if implemented too aggressively
- ✗ Complicates analysis

3. Arm Dropping

Multi-arm trial: Test 4 experimental arms vs control. Drop futile arms at interim analysis.

- ✓ Efficient — don't waste resources on non-performers
- ✓ Can reallocate patients to promising arms
- ⚠ Must pre-specify dropping rules

4. Biomarker-Adaptive Enrichment

Start broad: Enrol all-comers
Interim finding: Treatment only works in biomarker-positive subgroup
Adaptation: Restrict enrolment to biomarker-positive patients

- ✓ Can discover personalised medicine
- ✓ More efficient than separate trials
- ⚠ Risk of false-positive subgroup findings

Advantages vs Disadvantages

Advantages	Disadvantages
✓ More efficient	✗ More complex design/analysis
✓ Faster results	✗ Operational challenges
✓ More ethical	✗ Type I error inflation if not controlled
✓ Flexibility	✗ Difficult to interpret if many adaptations
✓ Can explore subgroups	✗ Requires sophisticated statistics

VIVA ANSWER:
"This is an adaptive trial with pre-specified interim analysis at 50% enrolment. The independent data monitoring committee can: (1) stop for efficacy if posterior probability >99%, (2) stop for futility if probability <10%, or (3) re-estimate sample size if effect smaller than expected. This design is more efficient than fixed design while controlling Type I error through Bayesian decision rules. The adaptation rules were pre-specified in protocol before any data collected, maintaining scientific rigour."

⚠ CRITICAL REQUIREMENT:
All adaptation rules must be:

- Pre-specified in protocol BEFORE trial starts
- Based on pre-defined decision rules (not data dredging)
- Reviewed by independent committee (not investigators)
- Control Type I error appropriately

Otherwise it's just post-hoc analysis masquerading as "adaptive"!

Card 10: Cluster Randomised Trials

What Is Cluster Randomisation?

Randomise GROUPS (clusters) rather than individuals

Examples of clusters:

- Hospitals
- Surgeons
- GP practices
- Geographic regions
- Time periods

Why Use Cluster Randomisation?

- **Contamination prevention:** Treatment in one patient affects others (e.g., hand hygiene intervention)
- **Intervention at group level:** Training surgeons in new technique — can't randomise individual patients
- **Pragmatic reasons:** Easier to implement intervention hospital-wide than patient-by-patient

- **Administrative simplicity:** All patients in one centre get same treatment

⚠ The BIG Problem: Intracluster Correlation

ICC (Intracluster Correlation Coefficient): Degree to which patients within same cluster are more similar to each other than to patients in other clusters.
Example: Patients operated by same surgeon have more similar outcomes than patients of different surgeons (surgeon skill, preference, technique)
Impact: Reduces effective sample size!

Design Effect & Sample Size

Design Effect = 1 + (m − 1) × ICC
where m = average cluster size
Required N = Individual RCT N × Design Effect

Worked Example

Standard RCT needs: 500 patients
Cluster design: 10 hospitals, 50 patients each, ICC = 0.05
Design Effect:
= 1 + (50 − 1) × 0.05 = 1 + 2.45 = 3.45
Required N:
= 500 × 3.45 = **1,725 patients!**
Need about 3.5× as many patients in cluster design!

Analysis Considerations

Method	Description	When to Use
Cluster-level analysis	Analyse cluster means	Small number of clusters
Individual-level with adjustment	Mixed-effects model	Many clusters, variable size
GEE (Generalised Estimating Equations)	Accounts for correlation	Complex correlation structures

✗ CRITICAL ERROR:
Analysing cluster RCT as if it were individual randomisation (ignoring clustering) produces:
- Falsely narrow confidence intervals
- Inflated Type I error
- Invalid p-values

Always check: Did authors account for clustering in analysis?

VIVA ANSWER:

"This is a cluster randomised trial with 20 hospitals randomised to an enhanced recovery protocol versus standard care. Cluster design is appropriate because the intervention requires hospital-wide implementation — you cannot have some patients on ERAS and others on standard care in the same unit, because of contamination. However, patients within a hospital are more similar to each other than to patients elsewhere, which creates intracluster correlation. The authors appropriately used mixed-effects logistic regression accounting for clustering at hospital level. With 1,200 patients across 20 hospitals — an average cluster size of 60 — and an ICC of 0.0085, the design effect is $1 + (60 - 1) \times 0.0085 \approx 1.5$. That is why they needed 1,200 patients rather than the 800 an individually randomised trial would have required."

✓ Reporting Requirements (CONSORT Extension)

- Number of clusters randomised
- Number of individuals per cluster (mean, range)
- ICC estimate and source
- Design effect calculation
- Method of accounting for clustering in analysis
- Cluster-level descriptive statistics

Card 11: Crossover Trial Designs

What Is a Crossover Design?

Each patient receives BOTH treatments in random order, serving as their own control

Classic 2×2 Crossover:

- **Group 1:** Treatment A → Washout → Treatment B
- **Group 2:** Treatment B → Washout → Treatment A

✓ Major Advantages

- **Increased power:** Within-patient comparison eliminates inter-patient variability
- **Smaller sample size:** Each patient contributes data for both treatments
- **Eliminates confounding:** Patient is their own control (same genetics, baseline risk)
- **Ethical:** All patients get both treatments (no one "loses")

⚠ Critical Requirements

Crossover design ONLY valid if:

1. **Condition is stable across the study periods**
   - ✓ Chronic pain, asthma, diabetes
   - ✗ Cancer (disease progresses)
   - ✗ Acute conditions (resolve before crossover)
2. **Treatment effects are REVERSIBLE**

- ✓ Medications (wash out after stopping)
- ✗ Surgery (permanent effect)
- ✗ Curative treatments

3. **Adequate WASHOUT period**
- Must eliminate carryover effects
- Five half-lives is a pharmacokinetic rule of thumb, not a universal requirement — washout must be long enough to minimise clinically relevant carryover, and pharmacodynamic effects can outlast the drug
- Long enough for outcome to return to baseline

When Crossover is INAPPROPRIATE

Scenario	Why Not?
Surgical interventions	Irreversible — can't "wash out" a hernia repair
Cancer treatment	Disease progresses; treatment order affects outcome
Training/education	Can't "unlearn" — permanent carryover
Cure or death outcomes	No crossover possible after cure/death
Long-term outcomes	Impractical to follow patients through both periods

Carryover Effects — The Big Problem

Period Effect:
Outcomes differ between Period 1 and Period 2 regardless of treatment

- Learning effects
- Disease progression
- Seasonal variation

Carryover Effect:
Treatment A influences response to Treatment B

- Incomplete washout
- Persistent side effects
- Psychological priming

Testing for Carryover

Compare **first-period data only** between groups:

- A difference in the first period is the treatment effect, which is why first-period data are used when carryover is suspected
- For carryover itself, compare subject totals across the two sequence groups (the Grizzle test)
- Can also test treatment × period interaction

VIVA ANSWER:

"This is a randomised crossover trial comparing two analgesics for chronic pancreatitis pain. Crossover design is appropriate because: (1) chronic pain is stable over the study period, (2) both drugs have short half-lives allowing complete washout in 2 weeks, (3) each patient serves as their own control, eliminating confounding by pain tolerance and baseline severity. The authors included a 2-week washout between periods and tested for period and carryover effects — both non-significant (period effect p=0.45, carryover effect p=0.38), validating the design. This increased statistical power, requiring only 60 patients instead of 120 for a parallel-group design."

⚠ **EXAMINER TRAP:**
"Why not use crossover for comparing laparoscopic vs open cholecystectomy?"
WRONG:
"Because surgery is irreversible"
RIGHT:
"Crossover is fundamentally inappropriate for surgical interventions for multiple reasons: (1) Surgery is irreversible — you can't 'wash out' a cholecystectomy and restore the gallbladder. (2) The condition being treated (symptomatic gallstones) is cured by first treatment — there's no opportunity for crossover. (3) Even if we could somehow reverse surgery, anatomical changes, scarring, and patient experience from the first procedure would create massive carryover effects invalidating the comparison. Crossover requires chronic stable conditions with reversible treatments — surgery meets neither criterion."

Analysis of Crossover Trials

- **Compare within-patient differences** (Treatment A − Treatment B for each patient)
- **Paired t-test** or Wilcoxon signed-rank test
- **Mixed-effects model** accounting for period, sequence, and carryover
- **Check for period × treatment interaction**

Card 12: Propensity Score Matching

The Problem It Solves

Observational studies have confounding: Patients who get Treatment A differ from those who get Treatment B in many ways (age, severity, comorbidities)
Goal: Improve balance in measured baseline covariates (this is not randomisation)

What Is a Propensity Score?

PS = Probability of receiving treatment
given baseline covariates
In plain English: How likely is this patient to receive Treatment A based on their characteristics?

How It Works — Step by Step

STEP 1: CALCULATE PROPENSITY SCORES

Use logistic regression:
Treatment (yes/no) = Age + Sex + Comorbidities + Severity + ...
This gives each patient a score (0 to 1) = probability of treatment

STEP 2: MATCH PATIENTS

1:1 Matching: Each treated patient matched to untreated patient with similar PS

Common methods:

- **Nearest neighbour:** Match to closest PS
- **Caliper matching: Match only if within 0.2 SD of the logit of the propensity score**
- **Many-to-one:** Match multiple controls to each treated

STEP 3: CHECK BALANCE

Compare baseline characteristics in matched groups:

- **Standardised mean difference (SMD) < 0.1** = good balance
- All covariates should be similar
- If imbalance persists → include in outcome model

STEP 4: ANALYSE MATCHED COHORT

Compare outcomes in matched groups:

- Paired analysis (since matched)
- OR Cox/logistic regression on matched sample
- Standard errors must account for matching

✓ Advantages

- **Controls confounding** by measured variables
- Creates balance in measured baseline covariates, partially emulating what randomisation achieves
- **Easy to explain:** "matched patients similar except for treatment"
- **Allows stratified analysis** by PS quintiles

⚠ Critical Limitations

✗ ONLY controls for MEASURED confounders!

Unmeasured confounding remains:

- Frailty (not captured in data)
- Surgeon skill/experience
- Patient motivation/compliance
- Socioeconomic factors

Propensity scores ≠ Randomisation!
RCT controls ALL confounders (measured + unmeasured)
PS only controls what you measured

Assessing Quality of PS Study

Check	Good Practice	Red Flag
Covariates included	All known confounders	Few variables, missing key factors
Balance assessment	SMD < 0.1 for all	Persistent imbalance
Matching quality	Narrow calipers, good overlap	Poor overlap in PS distribution
Sample loss	Most of the target population retained	A large share unmatched
Sensitivity analysis	Test robustness to unmeasured confounding	No sensitivity analysis

Alternative PS Methods

Method	Description	When to Use
Matching	Pair similar patients	1:1 comparisons
Stratification	Divide into PS quintiles, analyse within each	Maintain sample size
Weighting (IPTW)	Weight by inverse probability of treatment	Estimate population effect
Covariate adjustment	Include PS in regression	Supplementary to other methods

PERFECT VIVA ANSWER:
"This observational study used 1:1 propensity score matching to compare laparoscopic vs open liver resection. The propensity model included 15 baseline covariates: age, sex, ASA, tumour size, location, bilobar disease, neoadjuvant therapy, liver function, and comorbidities. After matching, 412 patients in each group had excellent balance with all standardised mean differences <0.08. This created balance in the measured baseline covariates, which partially emulates what randomisation achieves — but only for the covariates included in the model. However, unmeasured confounding remains — surgeon experience and patient selection factors not in database. The matched cohort showed significant benefit for laparoscopic (OR 0.68 for complications), but this should be interpreted cautiously given potential residual confounding. The ideal would be an RCT. Where randomisation is infeasible, well-conducted propensity-score methods improve comparability on the measured covariates, but they cannot balance unmeasured confounders and are not equivalent to randomisation."

⚠ **EXAMINER QUESTION:**
"Is propensity matching as good as randomisation?"
ANSWER:
"No. Propensity scores create balance on measured confounders only. Randomisation balances both measured AND unmeasured confounders — the truly random allocation means unknown factors (genetics, frailty, socioeconomics) are distributed equally. With propensity matching, if surgeon experience isn't in the database, it remains confounded. That said, when RCTs are infeasible (rare diseases, complex surgery, ethical constraints), propensity matching is our best tool for observational data. We should interpret with appropriate caution and look for consistency across multiple observational studies."

REFERENCE SECTION B: Critical Appraisal Checklists

Card 13: CONSORT Checklist (RCTs) — Essential Items

Title & Abstract

- Identifies as randomised trial
- Structured abstract with all key elements

Introduction

- Clear research question (PICO)
- Specific objectives/hypotheses

Methods — THE CRITICAL SECTION

TRIAL DESIGN

- Parallel, factorial, crossover?
- Allocation ratio (1:1, 2:1?)
- Changes after trial commenced?

PARTICIPANTS

- Eligibility criteria clearly defined
- Settings and locations
- Recruitment dates

INTERVENTIONS

- Detailed description (reproducible?)
- When and how administered
- Control/comparison described

OUTCOMES

- **Primary outcome specified**
- Secondary outcomes listed
- How and when measured

SAMPLE SIZE

- Power calculation provided

- Assumptions stated (effect size, alpha, power)
- Interim analyses/stopping rules

RANDOMISATION

- **Method of sequence generation** (computer, random number table)
- **Allocation concealment** (sealed envelopes, central randomisation)
- Block size (if applicable)
- Stratification factors

BLINDING

- Who was blinded? (participants, providers, assessors)
- How was blinding achieved?
- If not blinded, why not?

STATISTICAL METHODS

- Appropriate tests for data type
- **Intention-to-treat specified**
- How missing data handled
- Subgroup analyses pre-specified

Results

PARTICIPANT FLOW

- **CONSORT flow diagram** showing:
- Numbers screened → eligible → randomised
- Numbers receiving allocated intervention
- Numbers analysed (ITT)
- Reasons for exclusions/dropouts

BASELINE DATA

- **Table 1 — baseline characteristics**
- Groups should be balanced
- No p-values needed (it's randomised!)

OUTCOMES

- Primary outcome: effect size + CI + p-value
- Secondary outcomes reported
- Harms/adverse events

Quick Quality Assessment (original Cochrane risk-of-bias domains — superseded for RCTs by RoB 2, Card 15)

Domain	Low Risk	High Risk
Sequence generation	Computer/random table	Alternation, date of birth
Allocation concealment	Central/pharmacy/sealed opaque	Open list, unsealed envelopes
Blinding	Double-blind with placebo	No blinding, no justification
Incomplete data	Amount, balance and reasons	Substantial or imbalanced

Domain	Low Risk	High Risk
	reported; ITT with sensitivity analysis	missingness, reasons unexplained, per-protocol only
Selective reporting	All pre-specified outcomes	Outcomes added post-hoc

RAPID VIVA CHECK:
In 30 seconds, assess:
1. ✓ **Adequate randomisation?** (computer-generated)
2. ✓ **Concealed allocation?** (central/sealed)
3. ✓ **ITT analysis?** (all randomised analysed)
4. ✓ **Missing data handled well?** (amount, balance between arms, reasons, and method of handling — no fixed percentage decides this)
5. ✓ **Blinded outcomes?** (if feasible)
Do not convert this into a numerical score — name the domains that concern you and say why

Card 14: PRISMA Flowchart (Systematic Reviews)

What PRISMA Shows

Flow of studies through systematic review from identification to inclusion

The Three Phases (PRISMA 2020)

PRISMA 2020 replaced the older four-phase diagram. The separate Eligibility phase was folded into Screening, and the flow now distinguishes records found in databases and registers from those found by other methods. If you see a diagram with four bands including one labelled Eligibility, you are looking at the 2009 version.

- **1. Identification.** Records identified from databases and registers, and separately from other methods (citation searching, hand searching, contact with authors). Records removed before screening are shown here — duplicates, and anything excluded by automation tools.
- **2. Screening.** Records screened, then records excluded. Reports sought for retrieval, then reports not retrieved. Reports assessed for eligibility, then reports excluded with reasons. Note that the 2020 diagram separates the record you screened from the report you actually obtained — a distinction the 2009 version blurred.
- **3. Included.** Studies included in the review, and the reports of those studies. Where a meta-analysis was performed, the number pooled is usually smaller than the number included.

What to Say About It

Two questions earn marks. First, how wide was the net — how many databases, was grey literature searched, was the search restricted by language or date? Second, how steep was the drop — and were the exclusions at full-text stage justified? Excluded reports must be listed with reasons; if they are not, that is a reporting failure worth naming.

The gap between studies included in the review and studies included in the meta-analysis is where selective outcome reporting hides. If twelve studies measured an outcome and eight were pooled, ask what happened to the other four.

What to Look For

Check	Good Sign	Red Flag
Initial search	Multiple relevant databases, a reproducible search strategy with dates, and grey literature	A single database, no search dates, or unexplained exclusions
Screening	High number screened	Few screened (incomplete search)
Exclusions	Clear reasons documented	Vague/no reasons given
Final included	A number appropriate to the question	<5 (may miss evidence) >100 (too broad?)
Grey literature	Searched conference abstracts, registries	Published articles only

Example Numbers to Recognise Patterns

Well-Conducted Review:

- Identified: 3,247 records
- After duplicates: 2,156
- Screened: 2,156
- Excluded at title/abstract: 2,089
- Full-text assessed: 67
- Excluded at full-text: 45 (with documented reasons)
- **Included in review: 22**

Pattern: Funnel from broad search → selective inclusion. ~1% of initial records included.

Poorly-Conducted Review (Red Flags):

- Identified: 157 records (search too narrow)
- No duplicate removal mentioned
- Excluded: 140 (no reasons given)
- Included: 17

Problems: Incomplete search, lack of transparency, potential selection bias

VIVA ANSWER:

"The PRISMA flowchart shows a comprehensive search identifying 3,247 records from four databases plus hand-searching. After removing 1,091 duplicates, 2,156 were screened by title/abstract. The investigators assessed 67 full-text articles for eligibility, excluding 45 with documented reasons — primarily wrong population (n=18) and insufficient outcome data (n=15). Twenty-two RCTs met inclusion criteria for meta-analysis. This systematic approach with transparent reporting and high exclusion rate from broad initial search suggests comprehensive, unbiased study selection. The inclusion of grey literature search helps address publication bias."

Card 15: Risk of Bias 2.0 Tool (RoB 2)

Five Domains of Bias

The Cochrane **Risk of Bias 2 (RoB 2)** tool assesses risk of bias in randomised trials across five domains. Each is judged *low risk*, *some concerns*, or *high risk*; a single high-risk domain places the overall result at high risk of bias, as can an accumulation of some-concerns judgements that together substantially lower confidence. Note what is being judged: RoB 2 rates how much you should trust *this particular result*, not whether the trial was well conducted overall — the same trial can be low risk for one outcome and high risk for another.

1. Randomisation process

Was the allocation sequence random and adequately concealed? Do any baseline imbalances suggest a problem with randomisation?

2. Deviations from intended interventions

Did participants or carers know the assigned intervention, and did deviations beyond usual care affect the outcome? This is where intention-to-treat vs per-protocol sits.

3. Missing outcome data

Were outcome data available for nearly all participants, and could the missingness depend on the true outcome?

4. Measurement of the outcome

Was the outcome measured appropriately and outcome assessors blinded? Subjective outcomes judged by unblinded assessors are the classic concern.

5. Selection of the reported result

Was the reported result cherry-picked from multiple outcomes or analyses? A pre-registered protocol and analysis plan guard against this.

⚠ **Key point:** RoB 2 judges risk of bias *per outcome*, not once per study overall. The same trial can be low risk for its primary outcome but high risk for a secondary, subjectively assessed outcome — always specify which outcome you are assessing when using this tool.

VIVA ANSWER:

"I would assess this trial with the Cochrane RoB 2 tool across its five domains — the randomisation process, deviations from intended interventions, missing outcome data, measurement of the outcome, and selection of the reported result. Each is rated low risk, some concerns, or high risk, and a single high-risk domain — or an accumulation of some-concerns judgements — makes the overall result high risk of bias. Here the main concern is [domain], because [reason], so I would interpret the effect estimate with corresponding caution."
Reference: Sterne JAC et al. RoB 2: a revised tool for assessing risk of bias in randomised trials. *BMJ* 2019;366:l4898.

Checkpoint: the foundations are laid

You now have the toolkit: the sixteen chart types, the worked scenarios, the advanced statistical concepts, and the study-design cards. That is the material you draw *from*. What follows is where it comes together — and it is the half of the book that actually wins marks:

- → **Section 4** — the step-by-step framework that turns all of this into a structured verbal critique
- → **Section 5** — four landmark trials and a deliberately flawed paper, critiqued in full
- → **Section 6** — exam technique: the traps, the phrases, and what to do when you do not know

Keep going. The tools are only useful once you can wield them out loud.

SECTION 4: Step-by-Step Paper Critique Framework

One mental map for the reading period and the viva that follows

1 **Question** · What was asked? PICO.

↓

2 **Design** · Named in your first sentence.

↓

3 **Population** · Who was in — and who was left out?

↓

4 **Methods** · Randomisation, blinding, outcomes, power.

↓

5 **Bias** · Selection, performance, detection, attrition.

↓

6 **Results** · Effect size and precision, not just p.

↓

7 **Clinical significance** · Does the size of the effect matter?

↓

8 **Applicability** · Would it change practice — in your unit?

The first five ask whether the study can be believed.
The last three ask whether it should change anything.

In the viva

- Work in this order. A candidate who jumps to the result cannot defend it when asked why the design supports it.
- Steps 1–5 are about internal validity; steps 6–8 about what follows from it. Say which one you are answering.
- Do not reach step 8 without step 7 — a significant result too small to matter changes nothing.

Map 2 · The paper appraisal workflow — one mental map for the reading period and the viva.

4.1 The PICO Framework

Every research question can be broken down into PICO:
P = Population (who?)
I = Intervention (what treatment?)
C = Comparison (compared to what?)
O = Outcome (measuring what?)

EXAMPLE: CROSS TRIAL

- **P**: Patients with resectable oesophageal cancer
- **I**: Neoadjuvant chemoradiotherapy + surgery
- **C**: Surgery alone
- **O**: Overall survival (primary), R0 resection, pathological complete response (secondary)

4.2 Your Opening Statement

The examiner will say: "Tell me about this paper." You have 60-90 seconds to give a structured overview.

> Template:
> "This is a [study design] published in [journal] in [year] by [lead author et al]. The aim was to [research question in PICO format]. They [briefly describe methods]. The main finding was [primary outcome result with numbers]. This suggests [interpretation]. The key strengths include [one strength], but there are limitations such as [one limitation]."

EXAMPLE USING MAGIC TRIAL:

> "This is a randomised controlled trial published in the New England Journal of Medicine in 2006 by Cunningham and colleagues. The aim was to determine whether perioperative chemotherapy improves survival compared to surgery alone in patients with resectable gastric or lower oesophageal adenocarcinoma. Five hundred and three patients were randomised to either three cycles of ECF chemotherapy before and after surgery, or surgery alone. The primary outcome was overall survival. The trial found a significant survival benefit with a hazard ratio of 0.75 (95% CI 0.60-0.93, p=0.009), translating to a 5-year survival improvement from 23% to 36%. This represents a number needed to treat of approximately 8. The key strength is the pragmatic design reflecting real-world practice, but limitations include the heterogeneous population combining gastric and oesophageal cancers, and the relatively old chemotherapy regimen compared to current standards."

4.3 Methods Assessment Checklist

The examiner will probe your understanding of methodology. Be ready to discuss:

Study Population

- Who was included? (Inclusion criteria)
- Who was excluded? (Exclusion criteria — are they appropriate?)
- How were they recruited?
- Is the population representative of patients I see?

Randomisation (if RCT)

- How was randomisation performed? (Central randomisation? Computer-generated?)
- Was allocation concealed? (Did investigators know sequence in advance?)
- Was stratification used? (To balance important prognostic factors)

Blinding

- Who was blinded? (Patient, clinician, outcome assessor)
- If unblinded, is this justified? (Impossible in surgery often)
- Were outcome assessors blinded to reduce detection bias?

Interventions

- Are they clearly described? (Enough detail to replicate?)
- Were they standardised across centres?
- What was the control/comparison group?
- Were both groups treated identically apart from the intervention?

Outcomes

- What was the primary outcome?
- Was it clinically relevant? (Patient-centred vs surrogate)
- How was it measured? (Objective vs subjective)
- What were secondary outcomes?

Sample Size

- Was a power calculation done?
- Was the trial adequately powered for the primary outcome?
- Was recruitment target achieved?

Statistical Analysis

- Was it intention-to-treat or per-protocol?

- How was missing data handled?
- Were multiple testing corrections applied for secondary outcomes?
- Were confounders adjusted for in observational studies?

4.4 Results Framework

Patient Flow

Always review the CONSORT diagram (for RCTs) or flow chart:

- How many patients screened?
- How many randomised?
- How many received allocated intervention?
- How many completed follow-up?
- Reasons for dropout?

⚠ RED FLAGS:

- High dropout rate (roughly >20% — a warning sign, not a threshold)
- Differential dropout between groups
- Many crossovers between groups
- Large numbers not receiving allocated intervention

Baseline Characteristics

Check Table 1: Are the groups comparable? If there are significant baseline differences, consider whether this reflects chance imbalance (common in smaller trials), a problem with randomisation, or selection bias — and whether the analysis should adjust for the imbalanced variable.

Primary Outcome

This is the money question. You need to state:

1. The outcome measured
2. Results in each group (with numbers)
3. The difference between groups
4. P-value and confidence interval
5. Clinical interpretation

Example:
"The primary outcome was 5-year overall survival. In the chemotherapy group, 5-year survival was 36% compared to 23% in the surgery-alone group, representing an absolute difference of 13%. The hazard ratio was 0.75 with a 95% confidence interval of 0.60 to 0.93, and p=0.009. This is statistically significant and, more importantly, clinically meaningful — approximately 8 patients need to be treated to save one life."

Secondary Outcomes

Be brief but accurate. Examiners may ask about specific secondary outcomes, so scan them during your reading time.

4.5 Critique Structure

You'll be asked: "What are the strengths and limitations of this study?"

Strengths — Pick 2-3

Possible strengths include:

- Appropriate study design for the research question
- Adequate sample size and power
- Multicentre trial (improves generalisability)
- Good randomisation and allocation concealment
- Intention-to-treat analysis
- Low loss to follow-up
- Blinding where possible
- Clinically relevant primary outcome
- Long follow-up period
- Pragmatic design reflecting real-world practice

Limitations — Pick 2-3

Common limitations:

- Selection bias (strict inclusion/exclusion limiting generalisability)
- Single-centre study (limits external validity)
- Lack of blinding (detection bias)
- Short follow-up
- Surrogate outcomes instead of patient-centred outcomes
- Underpowered for subgroup analyses
- High dropout rate or differential dropout
- Outdated intervention (trial done years ago)
- Heterogeneous population making interpretation difficult

> **TOP TIP**
> Frame limitations constructively. Instead of just saying "there was selection bias," say: "The strict exclusion criteria may limit generalisability to elderly patients with multiple comorbidities who make up a significant proportion of our clinical practice."

4.6 Mock Viva Example: MAGIC Trial

Let's walk through a complete mock viva using the MAGIC trial as an example.

EXAMINER: "Good morning. Please tell me about this paper."

CANDIDATE:
"This is a randomised controlled trial published in the New England Journal of Medicine in 2006 by Cunningham and colleagues. The study investigated whether perioperative chemotherapy improves survival in patients with resectable adenocarcinoma of the stomach or lower oesophagus. Five hundred and three patients were randomised to either three cycles of ECF chemotherapy before and after surgery, or surgery alone. The primary outcome was overall survival. The trial demonstrated a significant survival benefit, with a hazard ratio of 0.75 (95% CI: 0.60-0.93, p=0.009). Five-year survival improved from 23% to 36%, representing an absolute benefit of 13%. Based on these results, perioperative chemotherapy became standard of care for resectable gastric cancer at the time, though it has since been superseded by FLOT for fit patients."

EXAMINER: "Good. What type of study design is this, and why is it appropriate?"

CANDIDATE:
"This is a randomised controlled trial, which is the gold standard for evaluating treatment efficacy. It's appropriate because it allows us to establish causality — that the chemotherapy itself improves survival, not just confounding factors like fitter patients choosing one treatment. Randomisation balances both known and unknown confounders between groups, giving us confidence that the observed difference is due to the intervention."

EXAMINER: "How was randomisation performed?"

CANDIDATE:
"Patients were centrally randomised using a minimisation procedure stratified by age, tumour site — stomach, oesophagogastric junction, or lower oesophagus — WHO performance status, and surgeon. Central randomisation ensures allocation concealment, preventing selection bias. Stratification ensures important prognostic factors are balanced between groups."

EXAMINER: "Was blinding possible in this trial?"

CANDIDATE:
"Complete blinding wasn't feasible since patients and clinicians obviously knew whether chemotherapy was given. However, this is less of a concern because the primary outcome was overall survival, which is an objective,

hard endpoint unlikely to be influenced by detection bias. If the outcome had been quality of life or symptom scores, lack of blinding would be more problematic."

EXAMINER: "Tell me about the baseline characteristics. Were the groups well balanced?"

CANDIDATE:
"Looking at Table 1, the groups appear well balanced. Age, gender distribution, tumour location, and stage are similar between groups with no significant differences. That balance is reassuring, though it is not proof that randomisation worked — randomisation is a feature of the design, and some imbalance is expected by chance whatever the process. What matters is that allocation was concealed."

EXAMINER: "Walk me through the primary outcome result."

CANDIDATE:
"The primary outcome was overall survival. The Kaplan–Meier curves show separation favouring the chemotherapy group starting around 12 months and maintained throughout follow-up. Five-year survival was 36% in the chemotherapy group versus 23% in the surgery-alone group. The hazard ratio was 0.75, meaning a 25% reduction in the hazard of death with chemotherapy — meaning at any given moment, patients on chemotherapy had 25% lower instantaneous risk of an event. The 95% confidence interval of 0.60 to 0.93 does not cross 1, so the result is statistically significant at the 5% level, consistent with the p-value of 0.009. Clinically, this translates to a number needed to treat of approximately 8 — meaning eight patients need perioperative chemotherapy to prevent one death at five years."

EXAMINER: "What are the main strengths of this trial?"

CANDIDATE:
"The main strengths are, first, the appropriate study design — an RCT provides Oxford Level 1b evidence — the highest individual-study level; a systematic review of RCTs would be Level 1a. (1a/1b are the 2009 Oxford labels, kept here because examiners still use them; the 2011 revision dropped the suffixes.) Second, the trial was adequately powered with 503 patients to detect a clinically meaningful survival difference. Third, it was an international multicentre trial — most patients came from 45 UK centres, with others in the Netherlands, Germany, Brazil, Singapore and New Zealand — which improves generalisability. Fourth, they used intention-to-treat analysis, which is conservative and reflects real-world practice. Finally, the primary outcome of overall survival is the most clinically relevant endpoint — it's objective, patient-centred, and what matters most to patients."

EXAMINER: "AND THE LIMITATIONS?"

CANDIDATE:
"There are several limitations. First, the population is heterogeneous, combining gastric, oesophagogastric junction and lower oesophageal adenocarcinomas, which may have different biology and chemosensitivity. That is partly by design: the trial opened to gastric carcinomas only and eligibility was widened in 1999 to include adenocarcinomas of the lower oesophagus. This makes it harder to determine which group benefits most. Second, by today's standards, the ECF chemotherapy regimen is somewhat outdated — we now use FLOT in many centres based on more recent trials. Third, eligibility required a WHO performance status of 0 or 1 — there was no upper age limit, but that fitness threshold still selects a population healthier than the patients we typically operate on, which limits generalisability to the frail and comorbid. Fourth, only 104 of the 250 patients assigned to chemotherapy completed all six cycles — 41.6% — and nearly half of those who got through the preoperative phase and surgery could not complete the postoperative half. The trial therefore tested a regimen most patients did not finish, which raises real questions about feasibility. Finally, although quality of life was a planned secondary endpoint, no quality-of-life results were reported in the primary publication, so we don't know the patient experience or the burden of treatment."

EXAMINER: "Would you change your practice based on this trial?"

CANDIDATE:
"Yes, this trial provides Oxford Level 1b evidence that perioperative chemotherapy improves survival in resectable gastric cancer, with a clinically meaningful absolute benefit. However, I would apply it thoughtfully. For a fit patient with resectable gastric adenocarcinoma, I would offer perioperative chemotherapy, though I'd use a more modern regimen like FLOT based on the FLOT4 trial. For an elderly patient with multiple comorbidities who would not have met the performance-status criteria for this trial, I'd have a careful discussion about the risks and benefits, as we don't have evidence in that population. For squamous cell carcinoma of the oesophagus I'd prefer neoadjuvant chemoradiotherapy based on CROSS; for adenocarcinoma of the oesophagus or GEJ, ESOPEC now favours perioperative FLOT. So the MAGIC regimen itself isn't what I'd use for oesophageal adenocarcinoma now — it's been superseded. So while this trial changed practice, it must be interpreted in the context of the individual patient and subsequent evidence."

EXAMINER: "EXCELLENT. THANK YOU."

SECTION 5: Practice Papers — Full Model Critiques

This section contains fully worked examples of landmark surgical trials, demonstrating how to structure your viva answers.

5.1 CROSS Trial — Oesophageal Cancer

Study Overview

Citation: van Hagen P et al. Preoperative chemoradiotherapy for oesophageal or junctional cancer. NEJM 2012;366:2074-2084. Long-term outcomes: Shapiro J et al. Lancet Oncol 2015;16:1090-1098.
Design: Multicentre randomised controlled trial
Population: 368 randomised (366 analysed, 2 withdrew) — resectable squamous cell carcinoma or adenocarcinoma of the oesophagus or gastro-oesophageal junction, cT1N0 excluded, ECOG 0–2, weight loss under 10%
Intervention: Neoadjuvant chemoradiotherapy (carboplatin/paclitaxel + 41.4 Gy) followed by surgery vs surgery alone
Primary Outcome: Overall survival

Key Results

Outcome	CRT + Surgery	Surgery Alone	P-value
R0 Resection Rate	92%	69%	<0.001
Pathological Complete Response	29%	-	-
Median Survival	49.4 months	24.0 months	0.003
5-year Survival	47%	34%	-

Model Viva Answers

> **OPENING STATEMENT:**
> "This is a multicentre randomised controlled trial published in the New England Journal of Medicine in 2012. It investigated whether neoadjuvant chemoradiotherapy improves survival in patients with resectable oesophageal or junctional cancer. Three hundred and sixty-eight patients were randomised, with 366 included in the analysis (178 chemoradiotherapy plus surgery, 188 surgery alone) to either chemoradiotherapy with carboplatin and paclitaxel plus 41.4 Gy radiation followed by surgery, or surgery alone. The primary outcome was overall

survival. The trial demonstrated a significant survival benefit, with median survival of 49.4 months in the chemoradiotherapy group versus 24 months with surgery alone (HR 0.66, 95% CI 0.50–0.87, p=0.003). The R0 resection rate increased dramatically from 69% to 92%, and 29% achieved pathological complete response. This trial established neoadjuvant chemoradiotherapy as an important standard treatment option for resectable oesophageal cancer, particularly squamous-cell carcinoma and historically for adenocarcinoma — a position subsequently refined by ESOPEC (2025) for adenocarcinoma (see Examiner Update below)."

STRENGTHS:

- "The study design is appropriate — an RCT provides Oxford Level 1b evidence (a systematic review of RCTs would be Level 1a)"
- "The primary outcome, overall survival, is clinically relevant and objective"
- "The trial was multicentre across eight Dutch centres, improving generalisability"
- "The chemoradiotherapy regimen is well-tolerated with manageable toxicity"
- "Long follow-up allows assessment of long-term survival"
- "High R0 resection rate suggests the regimen effectively downstages tumours"

LIMITATIONS:

- "The population was predominantly adenocarcinoma (about 75%), with squamous-cell carcinoma at roughly 23% and a small remainder of other histologies — consistent with Western practice. The point estimate of benefit was larger for squamous-cell carcinoma than for adenocarcinoma, but this is a subgroup comparison without a significant interaction, and the long-term report (Shapiro 2015) concludes the improvement is clinically relevant for both histologies. Quote it that way — reading a difference into non-significant subgroup point estimates is the error Chart N warns against"
- "The radiation dose (41.4 Gy) is lower than some other regimens, though this likely explains the better tolerance"
- "Surgical techniques varied — some patients had transhiatal, others transthoracic oesophagectomy — which may affect outcomes"
- "The trial excluded T4 tumours and certain patient groups, limiting applicability to more advanced disease"
- "Quality of life was not assessed, so we don't know the full patient burden of treatment"

Examiner Update (2024–2025): ESOPEC. The ESOPEC trial (Hoeppner, NEJM 2025) compared perioperative FLOT chemotherapy with CROSS-style neoadjuvant chemoradiotherapy in resectable oesophageal/GEJ adenocarcinoma, and found FLOT superior — 3-year overall survival

57.4% vs 50.7% (HR 0.70, 95% CI 0.53–0.92, p=0.01). So while CROSS established neoadjuvant chemoradiotherapy as a standard, current Level 1 evidence now favours perioperative FLOT for adenocarcinoma. (ESOPEC did not study squamous-cell carcinoma, where chemoradiotherapy remains standard.) Before transferring that result, note that ESOPEC enrolled a higher-risk population than CROSS: 6.6% were clinically staged T4 and 79.7% node-positive, against no T4 and 64.5% node-positive in CROSS. Pathological complete response was 16.7% with FLOT versus 10.1% with CROSS-style chemoradiotherapy — a secondary endpoint, so quote it as a descriptive difference rather than a demonstrated one. A strong candidate would acknowledge the shift when asked "has practice changed since this trial?" — and would say in the same breath that the two trial populations were not identical, which is the applicability question an examiner is waiting for.

Two further trials worth knowing. **Neo-AEGIS** (Reynolds, *Lancet Gastroenterol Hepatol* 2023) randomised oesophageal/junctional *adenocarcinoma* to CROSS-style chemoradiotherapy versus perioperative chemotherapy (MAGIC/FLOT). It closed early at its second interim futility analysis, after 143 deaths, on the basis of similar survival between the arms and the disruption of the COVID-19 pandemic — and found no significant overall-survival difference. Cite it as showing broad equivalence rather than superiority either way, noting that it had been converted to a non-inferiority design with a 5% margin. **JCOG1109 (NExT)** addressed the other histology: neoadjuvant regimens in *squamous-cell* oesophageal cancer. It was a three-arm trial — cisplatin/5-FU (CF) versus the docetaxel-containing triplet (DCF) versus chemoradiotherapy (CF-RT) — and DCF improved survival over CF. Naming all three arms is worth a mark: it shows you know the comparison was not simply "chemotherapy versus chemoradiotherapy." Taken with ESOPEC, the examiner-level point is that the question is no longer "chemoradiotherapy or not?" but "*which histology, which regimen?*" — adenocarcinoma has moved towards perioperative chemotherapy, while squamous-cell carcinoma remains a separate evidence stream.

CLINICAL APPLICATION:

"This trial established neoadjuvant chemoradiotherapy as standard for resectable oesophageal cancer, and it remains the standard for squamous cell carcinoma. For adenocarcinoma of the oesophagus or GEJ, ESOPEC now favours perioperative FLOT, so in that group I would offer FLOT to fit patients and reserve chemoradiotherapy for those unsuitable for triplet chemotherapy. Where I would still apply CROSS is squamous histology — where the pathological complete response rate was substantially higher than in adenocarcinoma. Within CROSS itself the benefit applied to both histologies and the interaction test was not significant, so the trial does not license me to withhold chemoradiotherapy from adenocarcinoma; what has changed is that a better comparator now exists for that group. I would be cautious about extrapolating to the frail or elderly patient: CROSS enrolled a fit population, so the trial does not tell me how such a patient will tolerate chemoradiotherapy. That is a generalisability limitation, and I would make the decision on assessed fitness in the MDT rather than on trial data that does not cover the patient in front of me."

5.2 MAGIC Trial — Gastric Cancer (Summary; full critique in Section 4.6)

(Summary only — the full model critique is in Section 4.6)

Quick Summary for Viva

Study: Cunningham D et al. NEJM 2006
Population: 503 patients with resectable gastric, oesophagogastric junction, or lower oesophageal adenocarcinoma
Intervention: 3 cycles ECF chemo before + 3 cycles after surgery vs surgery alone
Result: HR 0.75 (p=0.009), 5-yr survival 36% vs 23%, NNT≈8
Adjusted analysis: adjustment for the stratification factors, excluding surgeon, gave HR 0.74 (95% CI 0.59-0.93, p=0.008). A trial that minimised on surgeon could not adjust for surgeon: 129 surgeons across 503 patients leaves strata too sparse to fit as a fixed effect. Worth naming as a design-analysis mismatch.
Completion: 104 of 250 (41.6%) received all six cycles — the standard criticism of perioperative ECF, and a reliable examiner follow-up.
Impact: Established perioperative chemotherapy as standard of care

5.3 ACOSOG Z0011 Trial — Breast Surgery

Study Overview

Citation: Giuliano AE et al. Axillary dissection vs no axillary dissection in women with invasive breast cancer and sentinel node metastasis. JAMA 2011;305:569-575. 10-year outcomes: Giuliano AE et al. JAMA 2017;318:918-926. Locoregional recurrence: Giuliano AE et al. Ann Surg 2016;264(3):413-420.
Design: Randomised controlled non-inferiority trial
Population: 891 women with clinical T1-2 N0 breast cancer and 1-2 positive sentinel nodes
Intervention: Completion axillary lymph node dissection (ALND) vs sentinel lymph node biopsy (SLNB) alone

Primary Outcome: Overall survival, non-inferiority design with a prespecified margin of a one-sided hazard ratio of 1.3

Key Results

Outcome	SLNB Alone	SLNB + ALND	Comparison
10-year Overall Survival	86.3%	83.6%	Non-inferior (HR 0.85; one-sided 95% CI 0–1.16; P = 0.02)
5-year Disease-Free Survival	83.9%	82.2%	Not significantly different
10-year Locoregional Recurrence	5.3%	6.2%	No significant difference (p=0.36)
10-year Nodal (Regional) Recurrence	1.5%	0.5%	No significant difference (p=0.28)
Lymphoedema (subjective, 1 yr)	2%	13%	P ≤ 0.0001
Lymphoedema (arm measurement, 1 yr)	—	—	No significant difference

Overall survival is from the 10-year report (Giuliano, JAMA 2017); the recurrence rows are from the long-term locoregional recurrence report (Giuliano, Ann Surg 2016); disease-free survival is the 5-year figure from the primary report (Giuliano, JAMA 2011). Check the horizon and the source before quoting any single row.

The two lymphoedema rows are not a contradiction — they are the point. Subjective patient report showed 13% after ALND against 2% after SLNB alone. Objective arm measurement showed no significant difference. Same patients, same trial, opposite conclusion depending on how the outcome was ascertained. In a viva, "ALND causes more lymphoedema" is defensible only if you can say how it was measured. Source: Lucci A et al. JCO 2007;25(24):3657-63.

BOTTOM LINE

Z0011 was a non-inferiority trial, so its message is that sentinel node biopsy alone was not worse — not that the two are equivalent, and not that either is superior. In this selected population (T1-2, cN0, 1-2 positive sentinel nodes, breast-conserving surgery plus whole-breast radiotherapy), omitting completion axillary dissection did **not** compromise locoregional control, disease-free survival, or overall survival — while sparing the morbidity of ALND. The correct viva point is that SLNB alone is *non-inferior* to ALND for these patients; it is *not* that SLNB lowers recurrence. This does not extend to mastectomy, to more than two positive nodes, or to patients not receiving whole-breast radiotherapy.

Model Viva Answers

OPENING STATEMENT:

"This is a multicentre randomised controlled trial published in JAMA in 2011, with 10-year outcomes reported by Giuliano and colleagues in JAMA in 2017, investigating whether axillary lymph node dissection can be safely omitted in women with early breast cancer and limited sentinel node involvement. Eight hundred and ninety-one patients with clinical T1-2 N0 invasive breast cancer and 1-2 positive sentinel nodes were randomised to either completion axillary dissection or no further axillary treatment. All patients received breast-conserving surgery, whole breast radiotherapy, and systemic therapy. This was a non-inferiority trial — the hypothesis was that SLNB alone would be no worse than ALND, with a pre-specified non-inferiority margin of HR 1.3 for overall survival. At a median follow-up of 9.3 years, sentinel node biopsy alone was non-inferior for overall survival (86.3% versus 83.6%; HR 0.85, one-sided P = 0.02), and disease-free survival did not differ significantly. Non-inferiority is the claim the design supports: the trial shows SLNB alone was not worse, not that the two are equivalent. The trial concluded that completion ALND adds no demonstrable survival benefit and can be safely omitted in this population, potentially avoiding morbidity like lymphoedema."

STRENGTHS:

- "Pragmatic design addressing a clinically important question about de-escalation of surgery"
- "Primary outcome of overall survival is patient-centred and clinically relevant"
- "Well-conducted multicentre trial with good follow-up"
- "Results practice-changing, sparing patients from unnecessary morbidity"
- "Standardised adjuvant treatment in both arms ensures fair comparison"

LIMITATIONS:

- "Z0011 was a non-inferiority trial, with overall survival as its primary endpoint. It closed early because of slow accrual and a lower-than-expected event rate — an administrative early closure, not a formal futility stop — which limited its power to detect small differences, though it retained enough events for its pre-specified non-inferiority analysis."
- "Very specific inclusion criteria: only patients having breast-conserving surgery with whole breast radiotherapy, T1-2 tumours, and 1-2 positive nodes. Results don't apply to mastectomy patients or those with heavier nodal burden"
- "All patients received systemic therapy, which may have masked potential differences in axillary recurrence"

- "Tangential field radiation may have treated low axillary nodes, confounding the 'no axillary treatment' designation"
- "Longer follow-up might reveal late recurrences"

CLINICAL APPLICATION:
"This trial revolutionised breast surgery by showing we can safely de-escalate axillary surgery in selected patients. I would apply these results to patients meeting the exact trial criteria: clinical T1-2, 1-2 positive sentinel nodes, breast-conserving surgery with planned whole breast radiotherapy, and planned systemic therapy. For patients outside these criteria — for example, mastectomy patients or those with 3+ positive nodes — I cannot extrapolate these results and would discuss completion ALND. The key principle is that with modern systemic therapy and radiotherapy, microscopic nodal disease is likely controlled without surgery, sparing patients the morbidity of ALND."

5.4 Dutch TME Trial — Rectal Cancer

The classic examiner question: "How can radiotherapy reduce local recurrence without improving overall survival?"
A strong answer covers four points: (1) local recurrences are often *salvageable*, so preventing them does not necessarily prevent death; (2) patients still die of *distant metastatic disease*, which local radiotherapy does not address; (3) the trial can be powered for the recurrence endpoint yet *underpowered for survival*, where the effect is smaller and needs more events and longer follow-up; and (4) radiotherapy carries *morbidity* (bowel and sexual dysfunction), so the honest framing is a trade-off — fewer local recurrences at a real cost, without a proven survival gain.

Study Overview

Citation: Kapiteijn E et al. Preoperative radiotherapy combined with total mesorectal excision for resectable rectal cancer. NEJM 2001;345:638-646. Long-term outcomes: van Gijn W et al. Lancet Oncol 2011;12:575-582 — outcomes reported at 10 years, from a trial with 12 years of follow-up.
Design: Multicentre randomised controlled trial
Population: 1861 patients with resectable rectal cancer
Intervention: Short-course preoperative radiotherapy (5x5 Gy) + TME surgery vs TME surgery alone
Primary Outcome: Local recurrence rate

Key Results

Outcome	RT + TME	TME Alone	P-value
2-year Local Recurrence	2.4%	8.2%	<0.001
10-year Local Recurrence	5%	11%	<0.001
10-year Overall Survival	48.4%	49.2%	No significant difference (not evidence of equivalence)

Model Viva Answers

OPENING STATEMENT:

"This is a landmark multicentre randomised controlled trial published in the New England Journal of Medicine in 2001. It investigated whether preoperative radiotherapy reduces local recurrence when combined with total mesorectal excision surgery for rectal cancer. One thousand eight hundred and sixty-one patients with resectable rectal cancer were randomised to either short-course preoperative radiotherapy (5 fractions of 5 Gy over one week) followed by TME surgery, or TME surgery alone. The primary outcome was local recurrence rate. At 2 years, local recurrence was dramatically reduced from 8.2% to 2.4% with preoperative radiotherapy (p<0.001). This benefit persisted at 10 years (11% vs 5%). However, there was no significant difference in overall survival. This trial established short-course preoperative radiotherapy as a standard option for rectal cancer, though subsequent trials have refined patient selection."

STRENGTHS:

- "Large, adequately powered multicentre trial with 1861 patients"
- "Standardised surgical technique (TME) across all surgeons with quality control"
- "Primary outcome of local recurrence is clinically important and objectively assessed"
- "Long-term follow-up to 10 years shows the reduction in local recurrence is sustained — 5% versus 11% — with no overall survival benefit"
- "Short-course radiotherapy is practical and convenient (5 days vs 5-6 weeks)"

- "Pragmatic trial reflecting real-world practice"

LIMITATIONS:

- "The trial did not show an overall survival benefit, raising questions about the clinical importance of reducing local recurrence. The 10-year analysis does report better survival in TNM stage III patients with a negative circumferential margin, 50% versus 40% (p=0.032) — but that is a subgroup finding in a trial whose overall result was negative, and I would treat it as hypothesis-generating rather than practice-changing"
- "All patients received radiotherapy regardless of tumour stage — modern practice is more selective"
- "No long-course chemoradiotherapy arm for comparison"
- "Radiotherapy has long-term toxicity including sexual dysfunction, bowel problems, and secondary malignancies"
- "With modern MRI staging, we can now better select patients who truly need radiotherapy"
- "Early tumours (T1-2 N0) may not need radiotherapy, yet were included"

CLINICAL APPLICATION:

"The lesson I take from this trial is that quality TME surgery is what determines local control; radiotherapy reduces local recurrence but does not rescue poor surgery or a threatened margin. What has changed since is the staging, not that principle. I would stage with high-resolution MRI and stratify on MRF status, EMVI, nodal burden, tumour height and the relationship to the peritoneal reflection rather than on T and N alone. On that basis I would offer surgery alone for MRF-negative, EMVI-negative disease, and neoadjuvant treatment — short-course radiotherapy, long-course chemoradiotherapy, or a total neoadjuvant strategy — for higher-risk tumours, the choice depending on MRF threat, tumour height, fitness and whether organ preservation is being sought. I would add that the survival signal in the CRM-negative stage III subgroup was hypothesis-generating and the trial was not powered for it."

Interlude — A Messier Paper: The RPI Study

Teaching note. This is a constructed teaching case. No drug class called "renin pathway inhibitors" exists — treat RPI as a stand-in for any newly marketed, high-cost intervention. The numbers are invented but realistic, and every flaw shown here appears routinely in real database studies. The four worked critiques you have just read were deliberately clean, each isolating one idea. Real viva papers are rarely that cooperative. This one fails in three overlapping ways at once, and the skill being tested is not "spot the flaw" but "hold three flaws in mind at the same time and still give a calm, defensible verdict."

> ### Renin Pathway Inhibitors (RPIs) for Hypertension: A Cohort Study
>
> Journal of Clinical Hypertension (2024)
>
> **Background.** Renin pathway inhibitors (RPIs) are a recently introduced class of antihypertensive agents. We evaluated their association with all-cause mortality in routine clinical practice.
>
> **Methods.** Retrospective cohort study using linked NHS electronic health records, 2010–2019. 90,247 patients with a new diagnosis of hypertension were identified. Patients initiating RPI therapy were compared with those receiving standard antihypertensives (ACE inhibitors or ARBs). Primary outcome: all-cause mortality. We adjusted for 31 covariates using multivariable Cox regression.
>
> **Results.** RPI users had significantly lower all-cause mortality than standard therapy (12.3% vs 16.8%; adjusted HR 0.72, 95% CI 0.68–0.76, $p<0.001$). In a pre-planned subgroup analysis, the benefit was more pronounced in patients aged 75 and over (HR 0.61, 95% CI 0.54–0.69).
>
> **Conclusion.** RPI therapy is associated with a 28% reduction in all-cause mortality in hypertensive patients. This benefit appears particularly marked in older patients and should prompt reassessment of current prescribing practices.

Read on its own, that abstract is persuasive: a large study (N > 90,000), a hard endpoint, a big effect, a tight confidence interval, and a bonus finding in the elderly. A tired candidate reads "28% reduction in mortality, $p<0.001$" and starts nodding. Three things should stop you.

> Flaw One · Immortal Time Bias

The flaw	**"Exposure" was defined by filling an RPI prescription at *any point* during follow-up. To be counted as a user, a patient first had to survive long enough to reach that prescription. Anyone who died before filling it falls into the comparison group by default.**
The tell	The supplementary tables give the mean time from cohort entry to first RPI prescription: 4.2 months — 4.2 months of guaranteed survival handed to the RPI group before their "exposed" time even begins.
The direction	It inflates the apparent benefit. The window during which a future user cannot yet have died is "immortal." Attributing that survival to the drug makes it look protective when the design alone can produce the entire effect.
The fix	Treat exposure as a time-varying covariate; or run a **landmark analysis** — choose a fixed landmark (say 6 months), keep only patients alive and event-free at that point, classify them by their exposure status *at* the landmark, and start the survival clock there, so no one earns "immortal" time; or use a new-user, active-comparator design where every patient's clock starts at the same defined origin.

Why this one is decisive: an HR of 0.72 is well within the range that immortal time bias alone has produced in published pharmaco-epidemiology. You cannot tell how much of the 28% is drug and how much is artefact — and that is the point.

Flaw Two · Residual Confounding

The flaw	**The model adjusts for 31 covariates but not for frailty, functional status, cognitive impairment or care-home residence — precisely the factors that influence whether a clinician reaches for a newer, more expensive agent. Practice type was recorded, since it appears among the subgroups, yet it does not enter the adjustment.**
The tell	The paper presents "adjusted for 31 covariates" as a *strength*. Volume of adjustment is not the same as control of confounding.
The direction	Also toward apparent benefit — healthy-user, or treatment-selection, bias rather than classic confounding by indication, which usually runs the other way when sicker patients are preferentially treated. Fitter, better-attended patients are both more likely to be started on the new drug and more likely to survive. Adjustment removes the confounding you measured; it does nothing for the confounding you didn't.

Viva gold dust

"Adjusted is not the same as controlled. Multivariable regression can only correct for the parameters you actually thought to record. Only randomisation balances the invisible confounders."

Flaw Three · Multiplicity & the Subgroup Claim

The flaw	**Eleven subgroups were tested (age, sex, diabetes, CKD, prior CV events, deprivation, BMI, smoking, practice type, year of diagnosis, prior medication). The age-≥75 result was singled out for the conclusion.**
The tell	No test of interaction (p-interaction) is reported for age as an effect modifier. The abstract calls the analysis "pre-planned," but a pre-planned *subgroup* is not the same as a pre-planned *test of interaction*.
The direction	Toward a false positive (Type I error). With 11 independent tests at an unadjusted $\alpha = 0.05$, the chance of at least one spurious "significant" result is $\mathbf{1 - 0.95^{11} \approx 43\%}$. A striking subgroup finding is exactly what you would expect to appear by chance alone.

None of these three is fatal in isolation, arguably — but they do not sit in isolation. They all push the same way, and the first of them is strong enough to explain the whole result on its own. That is what "messy" means: not one clean error you can name and dismiss, but several partial errors that compound.

The Model Viva Answer

EXAMINER: "Walk me through this abstract and your evaluation of its conclusion."

CANDIDATE:

"This is a retrospective database cohort study of just over 90,000 hypertensive patients over a nine-year window, reporting a 28% reduction in all-cause mortality with renin pathway inhibitors — adjusted hazard ratio 0.72, p less than 0.001. It's a striking headline, but the design has three compounding flaws that together mean I can't rely on the conclusion: immortal time bias, residual confounding, and unadjusted multiplicity."

EXAMINER: "Take me through them. Which one drives the effect?"

CANDIDATE:

"The primary driver is immortal time bias. Exposure was defined by filling a prescription at any point in follow-up, and the mean time to that first prescription was 4.2 months. To be classed as a user, a patient had to survive those first 4.2 months — so the user group is guaranteed to be alive during that window, while anyone who died in it falls into the comparison group. That design feature alone can generate a hazard ratio of this size, independent of any real drug effect.

Second, residual confounding by indication. Adjusting for 31 covariates sounds robust, but adjusted is not controlled — they didn't capture frailty, functional status or practice type, which are exactly what decides who gets the newer drug. The fitter patients got the drug and survived because they were fitter.

Third, the over-75 subgroup. Eleven subgroups were tested with no interaction test reported. With eleven tests there's roughly a 43% chance of at least one false positive, so I'd treat that finding as hypothesis-generating, not a result."

EXAMINER: "So would you update your department's formulary on the strength of this?"

CANDIDATE:

"No. The honest position isn't 'prescribe' or 'don't prescribe' — it's that this study can't isolate a drug effect from the immortal-time artefact, so it doesn't give reliable information either way. The question is worth answering properly. I'd want a randomised trial, or at least a new-user active-comparator cohort with a fixed time origin, before this changed anything I do."

Notice what the strong answer does not do: it doesn't dismiss the paper as "worthless" (Section 6.4, TRAP 4), and it doesn't get lost trying to rescue it. It names each flaw, states the direction of each, identifies the one that is decisive, and lands on a calm verdict. That is the behaviour the viva rewards.

Ask Yourself

1. Can you name all three flaws *and* state the direction each pushes the result? (Here, all three push the same way — toward apparent benefit.)
2. Is immortal time bias a design flaw or an analysis flaw? Does the distinction change what could be done to fix it?
3. The subgroup analysis is described as "pre-planned." Does that alone make it trustworthy? What else would you need to see?
4. The residual confounding here can't be quantified from the paper. Does that make it less of a concern, or more?
5. How would you explain these limitations to a consultant about to change your unit's prescribing protocol on the strength of this abstract?

The consultation-room litmus test

When a retrospective database study claims a large survival or mortality difference, find the exposure definition in the methods before you read the results. Ask when the follow-up clock started for each group. If a patient had to survive to a milestone — or fill a prescription later in the timeline — to qualify as "exposed," hold the paper at arm's length. You are looking at a result that immortal time bias can produce on its own, and it should wait for a better-designed study to confirm it.

SECTION 6: Viva Checklists & Exam Technique

6.1 Complete Viva Checklist

Print this page and tick off items as you prepare. This is your final checklist before the exam.

✓ During the 30-Minute Reading Period

Timing	Task	What to Extract
0-4 min	Orientation (Pass 1)	Title, abstract, study design, main result, conclusion
4-16 min	Interrogation (Pass 2)	PICO, methods details, Table 1, main results table, p-values, CIs
16-24 min	Construction (Pass 3)	2-3 strengths, 2-3 limitations, clinical application
24-29 min	Rehearsal (Pass 4)	Opening summary rehearsed, first two answers ready, one number chosen

✓ Essential Elements to Identify

STUDY BASICS

- ☐ Journal and year
- ☐ Study design (RCT, cohort, case-control, systematic review)
- ☐ PICO (Population, Intervention, Comparison, Outcome)
- ☐ Sample size

METHODS

- ☐ How randomisation was done (if RCT)
- ☐ Blinding status
- ☐ Inclusion/exclusion criteria
- ☐ Primary outcome clearly stated
- ☐ Sample size calculation mentioned

RESULTS

- ☐ Patient flow numbers (screened, randomised, analysed)
- ☐ Dropout rate
- ☐ Baseline characteristics balanced
- ☐ Primary outcome result with numbers

- ☐ P-value and confidence interval
- ☐ Calculate ARR, RRR, NNT if possible

CRITIQUE

- ☐ Two major strengths identified
- ☐ Two major limitations identified
- ☐ Sources of bias considered
- ☐ Generalisability to my practice

6.2 Time Management Strategy

The 30-Minute Reading Period

> ⚠ **COMMON MISTAKE**
> Thirty minutes is long enough to read every word — which is exactly the trap. A candidate who reads the whole paper slowly arrives with recall but no argument. Use the four passes, and protect the last one: rehearsal is what the extra time buys you.

WHAT TO WRITE DOWN:

You'll have paper to make notes. Write:

- Study design and PICO
- Key numbers (sample size, results, p-values)
- 2-3 strengths
- 2-3 limitations
- ARR/RRR/NNT if you calculated them

During the Viva (15 Minutes)

Phase	Duration	What Happens
Opening	2 min	Your structured summary of the paper
Methods	3 min	Questions about study design, randomisation, blinding
Results	4 min	Interpreting tables, statistics, clinical significance
Critique	3 min	Strengths, limitations, bias
Application	3 min	Would you change practice? How does it apply?

6.3 Professional Language — The SBAR Technique

Structure your answers using SBAR (Situation, Background, Assessment, Recommendation):

Example: Answering "Would you change your practice?"

> **Situation:** "This trial provides Oxford Level 1b evidence for perioperative chemotherapy in gastric cancer."
> **Background:** "The absolute survival benefit is 13%, with a number needed to treat of 8, which is clinically meaningful in a disease with poor prognosis."
> **Assessment:** "However, the trial population excludes elderly patients with comorbidities who make up a significant proportion of my practice. Additionally, the ECF regimen is now superseded by FLOT."
> **Recommendation:** "I would offer perioperative chemotherapy to fit patients with resectable gastric cancer, using a modern regimen like FLOT. For elderly or frail patients, I'd have a shared decision-making discussion about the balance of benefits versus toxicity."

6.4 Common Traps and How to Avoid Them

TRAP 1: Confusing Statistical and Clinical Significance

> **Wrong Answer:** "The p-value is 0.001, so this result is very important."
> **Right Answer:** "The result is statistically significant with p=0.001, meaning it's unlikely due to chance. However, the absolute difference is only 1%, which may not be clinically meaningful. I would need to consider cost, patient preference, and quality of life before changing practice."

TRAP 2: Over-Interpreting Subgroup Analyses

> **Wrong Answer:** "The subgroup analysis shows benefit in patients under 65, so we should only treat younger patients."
> **Right Answer:** "The subgroup analysis suggests a trend toward benefit in younger patients, but this was not the primary analysis and may be due to chance given multiple comparisons. Subgroup analyses should be hypothesis-generating only and require validation in a dedicated trial."
> **Also know the converse:** a non-significant interaction does not prove the effect is uniform. These tests are usually underpowered, so it means the trial could not detect a difference — a weaker claim than showing there is none.

TRAP 3: Ignoring Limitations

> **Wrong Answer:** "This is a great RCT published in a top journal, so we should adopt this immediately."
> **Right Answer:** "While this is a well-designed RCT, there are important limitations including [specific limitations]. These affect how I would apply the results to my patient population. I would consider the trial evidence alongside patient factors and shared decision-making."

TRAP 4: Being Too Negative

> **Wrong Answer:** "This trial has too many flaws — selection bias, lack of blinding, heterogeneous population. The results are worthless."
> **Right Answer:** "Every trial has limitations, and this one is no exception. However, it provides valuable Level 1 evidence on an important clinical question. While I would be cautious about [specific limitation], the overall findings are informative and should influence practice when applied thoughtfully."

TRAP 5: Using Jargon Without Understanding

> **Wrong:** "There's selection bias because of the inclusion criteria."
> **Right:** "There's selection bias because eligibility required a specified performance status and fitness for the trial intervention. This limits generalisability because the trial population was fitter than the real-world population we operate on, and frailer patients may tolerate or respond to treatment differently."

TRAP 6: Quoting Kaplan–Meier When Competing Risks Apply

> **Wrong:** "The curve shows 40% recurrence at five years."
> **Right:** "That is a Kaplan–Meier estimate, which treats deaths from other causes as censored observations. That assumes censoring is non-informative; when competing deaths are common, Kaplan–Meier overestimates the cumulative incidence of recurrence. I would want a cumulative incidence function instead."

TRAP 7: Praising an AUC Without Asking About Calibration

> **Wrong:** "The AUC is 0.89, so it is a good model."
> **Right:** "The discrimination is good — the model ranks patients well. But AUC assesses discrimination, not calibration — it tells us little about whether the predicted probabilities are numerically accurate. A model can discriminate well and still tell a patient 89% when the observed rate is 66%. I would want to see the calibration plot before quoting a number in a consent conversation."

TRAP 8: Accepting a Non-Inferiority Margin at Face Value

Wrong: "The confidence interval sits within the margin, so non-inferiority is demonstrated."
Right: "It met the margin, but the margin is the appraisal. My first question is how it was justified — preservation of effect, clinical meaningfulness, and whether it was pre-specified. A margin that tolerates a clinically unacceptable loss makes the result meaningless however tight the interval."

Worked instance — Z0011 (Section 5.3). The margin was a one-sided hazard ratio of 1.3, pre-specified. The ten-year result gave HR 0.85 with a one-sided 95% CI upper limit of 1.16 — inside the margin, so non-inferiority holds. The appraisal question is whether a 30% tolerated increase in the hazard of death is clinically acceptable in this population.

TRAP 9: Forgetting Multiplicity

Wrong: "Pneumonia was significantly reduced, p equals 0.04."
Right: "That is one of four comparisons. Testing four outcomes at the 5% level carries roughly a one-in-five chance of at least one false positive. I would ask whether this outcome was pre-specified as primary and whether the threshold was adjusted — a Bonferroni correction here would require p below 0.0125."

TRAP 10: Confusing the Two Funnel Plots

Wrong: "The funnel plot shows publication bias."
Right: "It depends which funnel plot. One dot per study, assessed for asymmetry, addresses publication bias. One dot per unit against control limits is institutional outcome monitoring. They share a name and nothing else, so I would check which is being presented before commenting."

TRAP 11: Treating Crossing Curves as Proof

Wrong: "The curves cross, so proportional hazards is violated."
Right: "Crossing curves are a visual clue that the assumption may be violated, not proof of it. I would confirm formally with the Schoenfeld residuals test or a log-log plot. If the assumption genuinely fails, a single hazard ratio stops being a meaningful summary of the whole follow-up."

6.5 The Examiner's Fork — What the Question Is Primarily Testing

Examiners rarely ask what they appear to be asking. Most questions are a fork: one branch checks recall, the other checks judgement. Recognising which branch you are on is most of the work. The left column is what you hear; the middle is what is being assessed; the right is where a strong answer goes first.

If they ask...	Primarily testing...	Go here first
"How was the non-inferiority margin justified?"	Whether you recognise that justifying the margin is central to interpreting the trial	Preservation of effect, clinical meaningfulness, pre-specified
"The effect was larger in the elderly — comment."	Whether you reach for the interaction test or fall for subgroup p-values	"Is there a formal test for interaction?"
"The curves cross at 18 months."	Whether you can name the proportional hazards assumption	Schoenfeld residuals or a log-log plot
"The AUC is 0.89 — is this a good model?"	Whether you distinguish discrimination from calibration	"Good ranking — how does it calibrate?"
"Would you change your practice?"	Applicability, patient values and shared decision-making — not recall	SBAR, then your own population and its caveats
"40% had recurred by five years."	Whether you consider competing risks in an older or high-mortality cohort	Cumulative incidence, not Kaplan–Meier
"Pneumonia was reduced, p = 0.04."	Whether you notice this is one of several comparisons	Pre-specified primary outcome? Adjusted threshold?
"What does the funnel plot show?"	Whether you recognise which funnel plot is shown before interpreting it	Studies and asymmetry, or units and control limits?
"Is this result significant?"	Whether you separate statistical from clinical significance	"Statistically yes; clinically it depends on..."

If they ask...	Primarily testing...	Go here first
"Would these results apply to your patient?"	External validity, not internal validity	Trial population versus the patient in front of me
"The relative risk fell by 50%."	Whether you ask for the absolute benefit	ARR and NNT — and the baseline risk they depend on
"The secondary endpoint was significant."	Whether you notice it was not the primary outcome	What was the primary outcome, and was it met?
"What are the weaknesses?"	Proportion — balance, not a demolition	Two or three material limitations, then what it still shows

The pattern behind the fork. Almost every question above tests the same instinct: do you accept the number you are given, or do you ask what had to be true for that number to mean anything? Candidates who perform strongly usually move beyond naming the statistical test. They consider the assumptions, limitations and clinical implications before commenting on the result itself.

6.6 Phrases to Use and Avoid

✓ Powerful Phrases to Use

- "This provides Oxford Level 1b evidence that..." (or Level 1a for a systematic review of RCTs)
- "The absolute risk reduction is [X]%, which translates to a number needed to treat of [Y]"
- "While statistically significant, the clinical significance is..."
- "The confidence interval suggests the true effect lies between..."
- "This affects the external validity because..."
- "In the context of my clinical practice, I would..."
- "Balancing the benefits against the potential harms..."
- "This would inform shared decision-making with patients by..."
- "Was cumulative incidence reported, or is this a Kaplan–Meier estimate in a population with substantial competing mortality?"
- "The discrimination is good — how does the model calibrate?"
- "My first question in any non-inferiority trial is how the margin was justified."
- "Was that outcome pre-specified as primary, and was the threshold adjusted for multiplicity?"
- "Is that a formal test of interaction, or a comparison of subgroup p-values?"

✗ Phrases to Avoid

- Bluffing. If you don't know, say so and add what you do know: "I'm not certain of that figure, but the trial showed a survival benefit — I'd want to check the confidence interval." Honest uncertainty costs far less than invention.
- "The paper says..." (Instead: "The authors found..." or "The results demonstrate...")
- "It's significant" without qualification
- "Everyone should have this treatment" (too absolute)
- "This trial is rubbish" (too dismissive)
- "Obviously..." (nothing is obvious to examiners!)
- "The curves cross, so proportional hazards is violated" (overstates a visual clue as proof)
- "The AUC is 0.89, so it is a good model" (describes ranking only, not calibration)
- "It met non-inferiority, so it works" (skips the margin entirely)
- "It was significant in the elderly subgroup" (noise without the interaction test)
- "The funnel plot proves publication bias" — asymmetry does not prove it; small-study effects, heterogeneity, selective reporting and chance all produce asymmetry. Identify which funnel plot is shown, then describe what it demonstrates and what else could explain it.

6.7 Body Language and Presentation

PROFESSIONAL DEMEANOUR

- **Sit up straight** — project confidence
- **Make eye contact** — alternate between the examiners if there is more than one
- **Speak clearly** — don't rush, pause between points
- **Use your hands** — gesture naturally to emphasise points
- **Stay calm** — if you don't know something, say so gracefully

If You Don't Know the Answer

"I'm not familiar with that specific statistical test, but my understanding is that it's used for [general category]. Could you clarify what aspect you'd like me to discuss?"

OR

"Based on what I can see in the methods section, my reading would be [interpretation], though I would want to check that before relying on it."

6.8 Delivering the Answer Under Pressure

Knowing the content is not the same as delivering it. Three habits separate a candidate who knows the material from one who sounds like they do.

Lead with the conclusion

Examiners are listening for whether you can identify what matters. Give the answer in your first sentence, then support it. "This is a non-inferiority trial and its conclusion is that sentinel node biopsy alone was not worse — I'd want to check the margin and whether the population matches mine" tells the examiner more in ten seconds than a minute of describing the methods before reaching a view.

The recognition drills in this book are built for exactly this. What you see, what it means, key pattern — then the opener. Practise saying the opener first, not last.

The honest retreat

Bluffing is the one unrecoverable error: the examiner is a specialist and will see through it. But bare uncertainty wastes the question. Acknowledge the limit, then pivot to reasoning you can defend.

"I'm not certain of that specific figure. What I can say is that the confidence interval crosses one, so the trial has not demonstrated a difference — and I'd want to know whether it was powered to detect the difference that would matter clinically."

That answer concedes nothing you know and demonstrates the reasoning the question was testing. It is almost always worth more than a guess that happens to be right.

When the examiner pushes back

Repeated challenge is frequently a test of whether you will abandon a correct answer under pressure rather than a signal that you are wrong. Decide which is happening and say so.

If you can still defend your position: "I take the point, but I'd still say the analysis is complete-case rather than intention-to-treat, because 52 patients with no outcome data were excluded." If they have shown you something you had missed: "That changes my answer — I hadn't accounted for the imputation, and with it the analysis is intention-to-treat after all."

Changing your mind for a reason is a strength. Changing it because someone frowned is not.

Pace

> A two-second pause before answering reads as consideration, not hesitation. Rushing to fill silence is how candidates talk themselves into claims they cannot defend.

APPENDIX A: Quick Reference Tables

Study Design Comparison at a Glance

Design	Starts With	Best For	Result Measure	Evidence Level
RCT	Random allocation	Treatment efficacy	RR, HR, OR	1b
Cohort	Exposure status	Incidence, risk factors	RR, HR	2b
Case-Control	Outcome status	Rare outcomes	OR	3b
Cross-Sectional	Point in time	Prevalence	Prevalence ratio	4
Systematic Review	Multiple studies	Synthesising evidence	Pooled estimate	1a

Levels above follow the Oxford CEBM 2009 hierarchy, as in Section 1.3; both the 2009 and 2011 tables are question-specific, so the same design sits at different levels depending on whether the question concerns treatment, prognosis, diagnosis or prevalence; the 2011 revision dropped the a/b letter suffixes and reorganised the table. The levels quoted above are the treatment column. A cross-sectional study is Level 4 for "does this treatment work?" but sits far higher for "how common is this?" — read down the column that matches the question. Say why the evidence is strong or weak before reaching for a number.

P-Values and Confidence Intervals Quick Guide

P-Value	Meaning	What to Say
p < 0.001	Very strong evidence against null hypothesis	"Highly statistically significant"
0.001 0.01	Strong cvidcncc	"Statistically significant"
0.01 – 0.05	Moderate evidence	"Statistically significant at the

P-Value	Meaning	What to Say
		5% level"
0.05 - 0.10	Weak evidence	"Borderline" or "approaching significance"*
p > 0.10	Insufficient evidence against null	"Not statistically significant"

*"Approaching significance" legitimately *describes* a p-value of 0.05–0.10, but is spin when it implies a failed primary outcome succeeded — see §1.4 and Appendix E.

Confidence Interval Interpretation

Measure	Null Value	If CI Includes Null	If CI Excludes Null
Difference (means)	0	Not significant	Significant
Ratio (RR, OR, HR)	1	Not significant	Significant

Risk Measures Formula Card

Essential Formulas — MEMORISE THESE (ARR, RRR, NNT, RR, OR)

Absolute Risk Reduction (ARR):

ARR = Control Event Rate - Experimental Event Rate

Relative Risk Reduction (RRR):

RRR = ARR / Control Event Rate

Number Needed to Treat (NNT):

NNT = 1 / ARR

Relative Risk (RR):

RR = (a/[a+b]) / (c/[c+d])

Odds Ratio (OR):

OR = (a × d) / (b × c)

APPENDIX B: Statistical Tests Summary

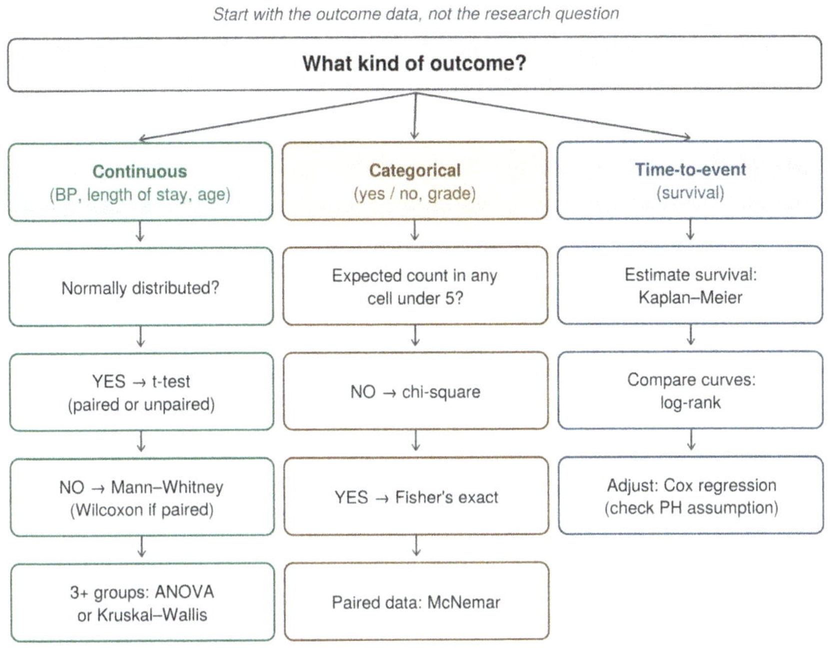

In the viva

- Name the test, then justify it from the data type — that is what earns the mark.
- Non-parametric tests are not inferior; they are correct when normality fails, and Fisher's exact is the right test for small expected counts, not a fallback.
- If they report a mean for skewed data, ask why a median was not used.
- Regression: linear for continuous, logistic for binary, Cox for time-to-event.

Colour separates the three outcome types only. No test shown here is inferior to another.

Map 3 · Which statistical test? Work from the outcome data type, then the distribution.

Choosing the Right Test

Scenario	Data Type	Normal Distribution?	Test to Use
Compare 2 independent	Continuous	Yes	**Independent t-test**

Scenario	Data Type	Normal Distribution?	Test to Use
groups			
Compare 2 independent groups	Continuous	No	**Mann-Whitney U test**
Compare 2 paired groups	Continuous	Yes	**Paired t-test**
Compare 2 paired groups	Continuous	No	**Wilcoxon signed-rank**
Compare 3+ independent groups	Continuous	Yes	**ANOVA**
Compare 3+ independent groups	Continuous	No	**Kruskal-Wallis**
Association between 2 categorical variables	Categorical	N/A	**Chi-square test**
Association: 2 categorical, small sample	Categorical	N/A	**Fisher's exact test**
Association: 2 categorical, paired data	Categorical	N/A	**McNemar's test**
Correlation between 2 continuous variables	Continuous	Yes	**Pearson's correlation**
Correlation between 2 continuous variables	Continuous	No	**Spearman's correlation**
Predict continuous outcome	Mixed	N/A	**Linear regression**
Predict binary outcome	Mixed	N/A	**Logistic regression**
Time to event analysis	Survival	N/A	**Log-rank test, Cox regression**

Statistical Test Selector — Visual Decision Tree

Choosing the Right Test: Decision Flowchart (a quick exam heuristic, not a substitute for checking assumptions)

START: What type of data do you have?

CONTINUOUS DATA (measurements)

Examples: Age, weight, blood pressure, operative time

How many groups are you comparing?

- └─ **2 groups (independent)**

– ├─ Normal distribution? → **Independent t-test**

– └─ Not normal? → **Mann-Whitney U test**

- └─ **2 groups (paired)**
  - ├─ Normal distribution? → **Paired t-test**
  - └─ Not normal? → **Wilcoxon signed-rank**
- └─ **3+ groups**
  - ├─ Normal distribution? → **ANOVA**
  - └─ Not normal? → **Kruskal-Wallis**
- └─ **Association between 2 variables?**
  - ├─ Both normal? → **Pearson correlation**
  - └─ Not normal? → **Spearman correlation**

CATEGORICAL DATA (groups/categories)

Examples: Gender, ASA grade, complication yes/no

Comparing 2 categorical variables?

- └─ **Paired or independent data?**
  - ├─ Independent, expected cell counts ≥5 in every cell → **Chi-square test**
  - ├─ Independent, any expected count below 5 → **Fisher's exact test**
  - └─ Paired (same patients, before and after) → **McNemar's test**

SURVIVAL / TIME-TO-EVENT DATA

Examples: Time to death, time to recurrence, time to discharge

- └─ **Comparing survival curves? → Log-rank test**
- └─ **Adjusting for covariates? → Cox regression**

Exam Shortcut:

1. Identify data type (continuous/categorical/survival)
2. Count groups (2 vs 3+)
3. Check if paired or independent
4. For continuous: check normality.

Understanding Regression Types

Regression Type	Outcome Variable	Result Interpretation	Example
Linear Regression	Continuous	For each unit increase in X, Y changes by β	Predicting length of stay from BMI
Logistic Regression	Binary (Yes/No)	Odds ratio for each predictor	Risk of anastomotic leak (yes/no) from age, smoking
Cox Regression	Time-to-event	Hazard ratio for each predictor	Time to cancer recurrence from stage, grade

APPENDIX C: Bias Types Reference

Comprehensive Bias Table

Bias Type	Definition	Example	Prevention
Selection Bias	Study sample doesn't represent target population	Trial enrols only fit patients but results applied to frail elderly	Broad inclusion criteria, consecutive patient enrolment
Performance Bias	Systematic differences in care between groups	Intervention group gets more clinic visits and support	Blinding of participants and clinicians, standardised protocols
Detection Bias	Systematic differences in outcome assessment	Assessors knowing treatment look harder for complications	Blinding of outcome assessors, objective outcome measures
Attrition Bias	Systematic differences in withdrawals	Sicker patients drop out preferentially from one group	Minimise dropout, intention-to-treat analysis
Recall Bias	Differential recall of past exposures	Patients with disease remember risk factors better than controls	Use objective records, prospective data collection
Publication Bias	Positive studies more likely to be published	Meta-analysis missing negative trials	Search grey literature, trial registries, funnel plots
Reporting Bias	Selective reporting of favourable outcomes	Highlighting secondary outcomes that are significant	Pre-registration of protocols, all outcomes reported
Lead-Time Bias	Early detection appears to improve survival without actually doing so	Screening detects cancer earlier, survival looks longer but death age unchanged	Use mortality as endpoint, not survival from diagnosis
Length-	Screening	Aggressive	Randomised screening

Bias Type	Definition	Example	Prevention
Time Bias	preferentially detects slow-growing cancers	cancers present between screens, making screening seem effective	trials, long follow-up
Observer Bias	Assessor's expectations influence measurements	Surgeon who performed novel technique assesses outcomes	Independent blinded outcome assessment
Hawthorne Effect	Participants change behaviour because they're being observed	Patients in trial comply better with treatment than real-world	Pragmatic trial design, minimal monitoring
Immortal Time Bias	Patients must survive long enough to receive the treatment, so the treated group is guaranteed early survival	Adjuvant chemotherapy appears to prolong survival because patients had to live long enough to start it	Landmark analysis, or time-varying exposure in the model
Confounding by Indication	The reason a treatment was chosen also predicts the outcome, so the groups differ at baseline	Unstable patients go straight to open surgery, making laparoscopic outcomes look better	Randomisation; if observational, propensity methods and explicit acknowledgement

APPENDIX D: Last 48 Hours Revision Pack

Revision Timeline Grid — Choose Your Strategy

Timeline	Phase 1	Phase 2	Phase 3	Phase 4	Phase 5
6-8 WEEK PLAN *(Comprehensive)*	✓ Section 1 (Foundations) ✓ 4-Pass Method ✓ Basic Statistics	✓ Section 2 (Study Designs) ✓ Section 3 (Statistics) ✓ Risk measures	✓ Section 4 (Framework) ✓ All Practice Papers ✓ Mock vivas	✓ Section 6 (Technique) ✓ Checklists ✓ Appendix C (Bias)	**APPENDIX D** **Quick Reference** **Viva Phrases**
2-3 WEEK PLAN *(Rapid Prep)*	**Days 1-7:** ✓ Speed-read Section 1 ✓ Focus on Section 3.2 (Risk Measures) ✓ Section 3.5 (Graphs) ✓ Master the Framework (Section 4)		**Days 8-14:** ✓ One Practice Paper per day ✓ Focus on your specialty ✓ Time yourself	**Days 15-21:** ✓ Memorise Section 6.1 (Checklist) ✓ Appendix A & B **Final 48 hrs: Appendix D only**	
EMERGENCY *(Last 48 Hours)*	*Not applicable — go straight to final 48 hours*				**APPENDIX D** + Quick Reference Card + One Practice Paper + Viva Checklist

Non-Negotiables (All Timelines)

1. **Risk Measures:** ARR, RRR, NNT (Section 3.2)
2. **Framework:** Step-by-step approach (Section 4)
3. **One Practice Paper:** From your specialty (Section 5)

Must-Know Trials by Specialty

Upper GI Surgery

Trial	What It Showed	One-Line Summary
CROSS	Neoadjuvant CRT for oesophageal cancer	CRT + surgery vs surgery alone: improved survival (HR 0.66, 95% CI 0.50–0.87), 29% pCR. Remains standard for squamous cell carcinoma; for adenocarcinoma see ESOPEC below
MAGIC	Perioperative chemo for gastric cancer	ECF chemo: 5-yr survival 36% vs 23% (NNT ≈ 8, derived from the survival difference, not reported by the trial). ECF now superseded by FLOT — see FLOT4 below
FLOT4	FLOT vs ECF/ECX for gastric cancer	FLOT superior: median OS 50 vs 35 months; HR 0.77 (95% CI 0.63–0.94)
ESOPEC	Perioperative FLOT vs CROSS-style chemoradiotherapy for oesophageal adenocarcinoma	FLOT superior: 3-yr OS 57.4% vs 50.7%; HR 0.70 (95% CI 0.53–0.92, p=0.01)

Colorectal Surgery

Trial	What It Showed	One-Line Summary
Dutch TME	Preop RT for rectal cancer	Short-course RT reduces local recurrence (11% → 5%) but no survival benefit
COLOR II	Laparoscopic vs open for rectal cancer	Laparoscopic non-inferior for oncologic outcomes
CLASICC	Laparoscopic vs open colorectal surgery	Laparoscopic safe and oncologically equivalent at long-term follow-up (an early signal of higher circumferential-margin positivity in laparoscopic anterior resection was not borne out on longer follow-up)

Breast Surgery

Trial	What It Showed	One-Line Summary
ACOSOG Z0011	Axillary dissection vs SLNB alone	Can omit ALND in T1-2 with 1-2 positive nodes having BCS+RT+systemic therapy
ALMANAC	SLNB vs axillary clearance	SLNB equivalent staging with less morbidity

HPB Surgery

Trial	What It Showed	One-Line Summary
ESPAC-4	Adjuvant chemo for pancreatic cancer	Gemcitabine + capecitabine superior to gemcitabine alone; now reserved for patients unfit for mFOLFIRINOX — see PRODIGE-24 below
PRODIGE-24	Adjuvant mFOLFIRINOX vs gemcitabine after resection	mFOLFIRINOX superior in fit patients: median DFS 21.6 vs 12.8 months, HR 0.58 (0.46–0.73); more toxicity

Statistical Concepts — Memory Joggers

The "Rule of 3s" for a quick approximate NNT (round up when you quote a final figure)

If ARR ≈ 3%, then NNT ≈ 33 (quote 34 if you are giving a final figure)
If ARR ≈ 10%, then NNT ≈ 10
If ARR ≈ 30%, then NNT ≈ 3.3 (quote 4)

> **CI Memory Aid**
> **Differences:** If CI crosses 0 → not statistically significant at the 5% level; the data remain compatible with no difference
> **Ratios:** If CI crosses 1 → not statistically significant at the 5% level; the data remain compatible with no effect
> **Width:** Narrow = precise; Wide = imprecise

Regression Quick Reference

- **Linear:** Continuous outcome (e.g., length of stay)

- **Logistic:** Binary outcome (e.g., complication yes/no) → gives OR
- **Cox:** Time-to-event (e.g., survival, recurrence) → gives HR

Final Checklist — Night Before Exam

✓ CAN YOU CONFIDENTLY EXPLAIN:

- □ The difference between RCT, cohort, and case-control studies?
- □ What ARR, RRR, and NNT mean and how to calculate them?
- □ How to interpret a p-value and confidence interval?
- □ The difference between ITT and per-protocol analysis?
- □ Three types of bias and how to prevent each?
- □ When to use Chi-square vs t-test?
- □ How to read a Kaplan–Meier curve?
- □ How to read a forest plot?
- □ The 4-pass method for reading a paper?
- □ PICO framework?

Emergency Phrases if You're Struggling

IF ASKED ABOUT UNFAMILIAR STATISTICS:

"I'm not intimately familiar with the details of that test, but my understanding is it's used to [general purpose]. The key finding here is [interpret the result shown]."

If asked to critique and your mind goes blank:

"Looking at this systematically — in terms of internal validity, [comment on randomisation/blinding]. For external validity, [comment on generalisability]. The statistical analysis appears [comment on power/appropriate tests]. If I were applying this to my practice, I would consider [patient factors]."

IF ASKED "WOULD YOU CHANGE PRACTICE?":

"This study provides [level of evidence] that [intervention] [improves/doesn't improve] [outcome]. The [strength] is [X], but I would need to consider [limitation] and [patient factors] before applying this broadly. For the right patient — [describe who] — this evidence supports [action]."

APPENDIX E: The Glossary of Spin

Most papers are written honestly. But when a primary result disappoints, the discussion section is where authors go to make the best of it — and there is a recurring vocabulary for doing so. Learning to hear what a phrase is *not* saying is one of the most quickly rewarded skills in the viva room. This is not a charge sheet against researchers; it is a translation guide. A good paper that hedges transparently will survive every entry below. Your task is to notice when the hedge is doing concealment work.

1 · When the primary outcome failed

What the paper says	The viva translation
"The treatment showed a trend towards significance."	The primary outcome was not significant. "Trend" is the word authors reach for when they cannot write "significant."
"The primary endpoint was not met; however..."	Stop at "however." Everything after it is hypothesis generation dressed as a finding.
"In a pre-specified secondary analysis..."	The primary analysis failed; this is what turned up next. A genuinely pre-specified secondary can be a legitimate signal — but it cannot carry the weight of a failed primary, and here it is being asked to.
"Although not statistically significant, the effect was clinically meaningful."	The threshold for "meaningful" appears to have been decided after the result was seen.
"We cannot rule out a type II error."	The study was underpowered (a type II, or β, error). The authors would like you to believe the drug works despite the data.
"There was no significant difference in the primary outcome."	It didn't work for the main thing. The paragraphs that follow will be about the secondary outcomes.
"Further studies are needed."	We could not prove our hypothesis. Someone should try again — ideally funding us. (Occasionally, though, it is simply true.)

2 · When the statistics are being nudged

What the paper says	The viva translation
"We adjusted for 47 covariates."	Volume of adjustment is offered as reassurance. Adjusted is not controlled, and enough covariates create room to find the model that best fit the story.
"Sensitivity analysis confirmed the primary result."	Sometimes reassuring. Sometimes several analyses were run and the one that agreed is the one reported — ask how many, and which.
"The confidence interval excluded the null value."	Occasionally the bound sits at 0.99 — technically significant, clinically indistinguishable from no effect. Read the whole interval, not just which side of the line it lands.
"We performed a post-hoc power calculation."	Power calculated from the observed effect of a study that has already failed just re-expresses the p-value. It tells you nothing you didn't already know.
"The effect was consistent across all subgroups."	Often the subgroup intervals were so wide that none of them could have disagreed with the overall result.
"We used a per-protocol analysis."	The patients who couldn't tolerate the treatment were excluded — which flatters the result. Ask for the intention-to-treat figure.
"Small but statistically significant."	Real, but probably too small to change what you do for the patient in front of you.

3 · When generalisability is being oversold

What the paper says	The viva translation
"Baseline characteristics were well balanced."	The *measured* characteristics were similar. In an observational study, the unmeasured ones may not have been.
"This multicentre study enhances generalisability."	Sometimes a genuine strength. But multiple centres also mean multiple local protocols and variable adherence — read it as a question to ask, not a guarantee.
"This is a pragmatic trial reflecting real-world practice."	Sometimes exactly the right design. Sometimes a loosely standardised intervention with a lot of missing data, framed as a design choice rather

What the paper says	The viva translation
	than a limitation.
"Real-world effectiveness is likely to be similar."	There is no real-world data yet. This is an aspiration.
"The study population was representative."	It resembled the patients who happened to be available at the participating sites.
"Our findings are consistent with the existing literature."	Consistent with the positive literature. The negative or equivocal studies tend not to reach the discussion section.
"This study adds to the growing body of evidence."	The growing body of evidence is sometimes the same group's earlier work.

4 · When safety and durability are being stretched

What the paper says	The viva translation
"Long-term safety data are reassuring."	Check the follow-up. "Long-term" frequently means 12–24 months.
"The trial was stopped early for overwhelming efficacy."	An interim analysis crossed a stopping boundary. Effect sizes at early stopping tend to overestimate the truth, and stopped trials capture fewer late harms.
"Open-label extension studies suggest durability of effect."	The patients who responded and tolerated the drug stayed on it. Those who didn't have already left the analysis — survivorship, not durability.
"All patients received standard care."	What "standard care" actually was is usually unspecified and unverified.
"We used a validated patient-reported outcome measure."	The endpoint is what the patient reports — which matters greatly if the patient knew their allocation and the trial wasn't blinded.

5 · When the framing is doing the persuading

What the paper says	The viva translation
"This is the largest study of its kind."	Sometimes genuinely important. Sometimes no one else had thought the question worth studying.
"This is a hypothesis-	We found something we can't yet prove and would

What the paper says	The viva translation
generating study."	like resources to pursue it.
"The authors are recognised experts in the field."	Irrelevant to whether allocation was concealed or the outcome pre-specified. Judge the paper, not the pedigree.
"Patients were randomised."	Reassuring only if the paper says *how* the sequence was generated and whether allocation was concealed. "Randomised" without a method is a claim, not evidence.
"A number needed to treat of X compares favourably."	Compared with what? An NNT means little without the comparator, the baseline risk, and the time horizon it was calculated over.
"The results were highly significant ($p<0.001$)."	A very small p-value in a very large study can attach to a difference far too small to matter. Significance is not size.

Morgan's caution — not every hedge is spin

Read this glossary as a set of prompts, not verdicts. "Further research is needed" is sometimes the most honest sentence in a paper. A pre-specified secondary analysis can be a genuinely valuable signal. A pragmatic trial's loose standardisation may be exactly right for the question. The skill is not to sneer at every cautious phrase — it is to notice when caution is being used to slide a failed result past you, and to say so precisely. In the viva, the phrase that scores is never a lazy "this is spin." It is: **"the authors describe X as a strength; I would read it as a limitation, because..."**

Cross-references. The mechanics behind these translations are covered in Section 1.4 (p-values and confidence intervals), Section 3.2 (risk measures), Section 4.3 (subgroup analysis and multiplicity), and the Advanced Modules (multiple testing; publication bias). Immortal time bias — the flaw behind several database-study claims — is worked through in full in the Messy Paper interlude at the end of Section 5.

APPENDIX F: Test Yourself

Eight abstracts, eight flaws. Each of these is a constructed teaching case — the study names are invented and the numbers are illustrative — but every flaw is one the FRCS academic viva loves to test. Read the abstract, decide the single most important weakness before you read the model answer that follows it, and practise saying your verdict out loud in one or two sentences. The examiner is not testing whether you can list ten limitations; they are testing whether you can name the one that matters and defend it calmly.

Exercise 1

Abstract · GLIDE trial
420 patients with symptomatic peripheral arterial disease were randomised to drug-eluting versus bare-metal stents. The primary endpoint was angiographic late lumen loss at 12 months. Drug-eluting stents showed significantly less late lumen loss (0.3 mm vs 0.9 mm, $p<0.001$). The authors conclude that drug-eluting stents "should be the preferred option for this population."

What is the single most important weakness?

Model answer

Surrogate endpoint. Late lumen loss is an angiographic surrogate, not a patient-important outcome. A stent can look better on imaging without the patient walking further, keeping their limb, or avoiding re-intervention.
"The primary endpoint here is a surrogate — late lumen loss — not a clinical outcome. I'd want to see this powered for amputation-free survival, re-intervention, or walking distance before I changed practice, because surrogate improvements don't reliably translate into patient benefit."

Exercise 2

Abstract · SHORT trial
A non-inferiority RCT randomised 600 patients with intra-abdominal infection to a 3-day versus a 7-day antibiotic course, with a non-inferiority margin of 10% for treatment failure. In the per-protocol analysis, treatment failure was 12% (3-day) vs 11% (7-day), a difference of 1% (95% CI −4% to +6%), within the margin. The authors conclude the short

course is "non-inferior." An intention-to-treat analysis is not reported as a primary result.

What is the single most important weakness?

Model answer

Reliance on a single analysis in a non-inferiority trial. Non-inferiority must be demonstrated in *both* the intention-to-treat and per-protocol analyses. ITT tends to bias *towards* non-inferiority by diluting the groups toward one another, and per-protocol breaks randomisation — so neither alone is sufficient. Reporting only the per-protocol result leaves the claim unsupported.

"This is a non-inferiority trial resting on per-protocol analysis alone. Per-protocol breaks randomisation; ITT dilutes the groups towards one another and so tends to favour a non-inferiority claim. Neither is safe by itself — I would want the two analyses to agree before accepting that a 3-day course is genuinely non-inferior."

Exercise 3

Abstract · CARE trial

1,200 patients were randomised to a new anticoagulant versus standard care. The primary outcome was a composite of death, myocardial infarction, stroke, or hospitalisation for a bleeding event. The composite occurred in 18% versus 23% (p=0.03). The authors conclude the drug "reduces cardiovascular events."

What is the single most important weakness?

Model answer

Composite endpoint — need the component breakdown. A composite is only as trustworthy as its parts. If the difference is driven by the softest, most frequent component (here, hospitalisation for bleeding) while the hard outcomes — death, MI, stroke — don't move, the headline overstates the benefit. The direction is also worth interrogating: counting a bleeding event as part of a "cardiovascular benefit" for an anticoagulant needs scrutiny.

"I'd want the individual components before accepting 'reduces cardiovascular events.' A composite driven by its least serious element can look impressive while the outcomes that matter most are unchanged."

Exercise 4

> **Abstract · REST trial**
> 80 patients with mild gallstone pancreatitis were randomised to early versus delayed cholecystectomy. Thirty-day complications occurred in 15% versus 22% (p=0.39). The authors conclude there is "no difference between early and delayed surgery."

What is the single most important weakness?

Model answer

Underpowered — absence of evidence is not evidence of absence. With only 80 patients, the trial cannot exclude a clinically important difference; a 7% absolute gap with p=0.39 is exactly what an underpowered study looks like (a wide, uninformative confidence interval). "No difference" should be "we did not detect a difference."

"This is a negative result, not a null result. The study is too small to exclude a meaningful difference, so I'd say it failed to detect a difference rather than that none exists — and I'd want the confidence interval and the power calculation."

Exercise 5

> **Abstract · BEAM trial**
> 900 patients with resected gastric cancer were randomised to adjuvant therapy versus placebo. The primary outcome, overall survival, showed HR 0.94 (95% CI 0.80–1.10) — not significant. In a pre-specified subgroup of node-positive patients, HR was 0.78 (95% CI 0.62–0.98, p=0.03). The authors recommend adjuvant therapy "for node-positive patients."

What is the single most important weakness?

Model answer

A positive subgroup rescuing a failed primary. The trial was negative overall. A subgroup result — even a pre-specified one — cannot carry the weight of a failed primary outcome, and with multiple subgroups tested the chance of a spurious "significant" one is high. This is hypothesis-generating, not practice-changing.

"The primary endpoint was negative, so I'd treat the node-positive subgroup as hypothesis-generating only. Pre-specification helps, but it doesn't turn a failed trial into a positive one — this needs a dedicated confirmatory trial before I'd recommend it."

Exercise 6

Abstract · registry cohort
In a registry of 3,000 patients with resected colorectal cancer, those who received adjuvant chemotherapy had better 5-year survival than those who did not (72% vs 61%, p<0.001). The authors conclude that chemotherapy "improves survival in routine practice."

What is the single most important weakness?

Model answer

Immortal time bias (plus confounding by indication). Patients had to survive long enough — and be well enough — to start chemotherapy; that guaranteed early survival time is "immortal" and inflates the treated group's apparent benefit. On top of that, fitter patients are selected for chemotherapy. This is observational data masquerading as an effect.
"This is immortal time bias: you can't die before you start treatment, so the treated group looks better for a reason that has nothing to do with the drug. Add confounding by indication and the survival gap is largely artefact — I'd want a landmark or time-dependent analysis, and really an RCT."

Exercise 7

Abstract · observational series
In an observational study of 5,000 emergency laparotomies, the laparoscopic approach was associated with lower 30-day mortality than open surgery (2% vs 8%, p<0.001). The authors conclude that laparoscopy "is safer for emergency surgery."

What is the single most important weakness?

Model answer

Confounding by indication. The groups are not comparable at baseline: the unstable, contaminated, physiologically deranged patient goes straight to an open operation, while the laparoscopic route is chosen for the more stable patient. The mortality difference reflects who was selected for each approach, not the approach itself.
"This is confounding by indication — sicker patients were selected for open surgery, so the comparison isn't fair. You can't conclude laparoscopy

is safer from observational data where the sickest patients were never eligible for it."

Exercise 8

Abstract · MARGIN trial

A non-inferiority RCT compared a new graft with the standard graft for elective aneurysm repair. The non-inferiority margin for 30-day mortality was set at 15% (absolute). Mortality was 9% with the new graft versus 4% with standard, a difference of 5% (95% CI −1% to +11%), within the 15% margin — so the authors declare the new graft "non-inferior."

What is the single most important weakness?

Model answer

An indefensibly wide non-inferiority margin. A margin that tolerates up to a 15% absolute increase in mortality can label a clearly worse device "non-inferior." The margin is the whole appraisal: if it is set too generously, the conclusion is meaningless. Here the point estimate already shows mortality more than doubling.

"The first question in any non-inferiority trial is how the margin was justified. A 15% mortality margin is clinically unacceptable — it lets a graft that doubles mortality pass as 'non-inferior.' I wouldn't accept the conclusion regardless of the confidence interval."

These eight cover the flaws most often tested: surrogate endpoints, single-analysis reliance in non-inferiority, composite endpoints, underpowering, subgroup rescue, immortal time bias, confounding by indication, and margin justification. Constructed teaching cases.

Index

2×2 Contingency Tables - Chart D (Section 3.5)
4-Pass Method - Section 1.2
Absolute Risk Reduction (ARR) - Section 3.2, Chart D
ACOSOG Z0011 Trial - Section 5.3
Adaptive Trial Designs - Card 9
Agreement vs Correlation - Chart P
ANOVA - Section 3.1, Appendix B
Area Under Curve (AUC) - Chart H (ROC Curves)
Attrition Bias - Section 1.5, Appendix C
Bar Charts - Chart C (Section 3.5)
Baseline Characteristics - Section 4.4
Bayesian vs Frequentist - Card 8
Bias Types - Section 1.5, Appendix C
Bland–Altman Plots - Chart P (Section 3.5)
Blinding - Section 1.3, 2.3, 4.3
Bonferroni Correction - Card 4, Chart C, Section 6.4 (TRAP 9)
Box Plots (Box-and-Whisker) - Chart F (Section 3.5)
Calibration (risk models) - Chart M
Case-Control Studies - Section 2.2
Chi-square Test - Section 3.1, Appendix B
Clinical Significance - Section 1.4, 3.2
Cluster Randomised Trials - Card 10
Cohort Studies - Section 1.3, 2.2
Competing Risks - Section 3.5, Chart L, Card 6, Section 6.4 (TRAP 6)
Confidence Intervals (CI) - Section 1.4, Appendix A
Confounding - Section 1.5, Card 5
CONSORT Checklist - Card 13
CONSORT Diagram - Section 4.4, Chart J
Correlation Coefficient (r) - Chart G (Scatter Plots)
Cox Regression - Section 3.3, Appendix B
CROSS Trial - Section 5.1, Appendix D
Crossover Trial Designs - Card 11
Cumulative Incidence Function - Chart L
Detection Bias - Section 1.5, Appendix C
Dutch TME Trial - Section 5.4, Appendix D
Effect Modification - Card 5, Chart N
ESOPEC Trial - Section 5.1, Introduction, References
Evidence Hierarchy - Section 1.3
Fisher's Exact Test - Section 3.1, Appendix B
FLOT / FLOT4 - Section 4.6, Section 5.1, Section 6.3, Appendix D
Forest Plots - Chart B (Section 3.5)
Funnel Plot (institutional audit) - Chart O

Funnel Plots - Chart I (Section 3.5)
Hazard Ratio - Section 1.4, Card 6
Heterogeneity (I^2) - Section 2.4, Chart B
Hypothesis Testing - Section 1.4
Immortal Time Bias - Interlude (RPI Study), Appendix C, Appendix F Ex 6
Intention-to-Treat - Section 2.3, 4.3, Card 3
Interquartile Range (IQR) - Chart F (Box Plots)
Kaplan–Meier Curves - Chart A (Section 3.5)
Lead-Time Bias - Module 1 Example 3, Appendix C
Limits of Agreement - Chart P
Logistic Regression - Section 3.3, Appendix B
MAGIC Trial - Section 4.6, 5.2, Appendix D
Mann-Whitney U Test - Section 3.1, Appendix B
Median - Chart F (Box Plots)
Meta-Analysis - Section 2.4
Multiplicity - Section 6.4 (TRAP 9), Card 4, Chart C, Chart N
NNH (Number Needed to Harm) - Section 3.2, Chart D, Module 1 Example 1
Non-Inferiority Trials - Section 5.3, Section 6.4 (TRAP 8), Card 2, Card 3, Appendix F Ex 2, Ex 8
Normal Distribution - Section 3.1
Number Needed to Treat (NNT) - Section 3.2, Chart D, Appendix A
Odds Ratio - Section 2.2, Chart D, Appendix A
P-Values - Section 1.4, Appendix A
Performance Bias - Section 1.5, Appendix C
PICO Framework - Section 4.1
Pie Charts - Chart E (Section 3.5)
Power Calculation - Section 4.3
PRISMA Diagram - Chart K
PRISMA Flowchart - Card 14, Chart K
PRODIGE-24 Trial - References, Appendix D
Propensity Score Matching - Card 12, Appendix C
Proportional Hazards Assumption - Card 1, Card 6, Section 6.4 (TRAP 11), Chart A
Publication Bias - Chart I (Funnel Plots), Appendix C
Publication Bias - Detection - Card 7, Chart I
Randomisation - Section 1.3, 2.3, 4.3
Randomised Controlled Trials - Section 1.3, 2.3
Recall Bias - Appendix C
Regression Analysis - Section 3.3, Appendix B
Relative Risk - Section 2.2, Appendix A
Relative Risk Reduction (RRR) - Section 3.2, Appendix A
Risk of Bias 2 (RoB 2) - Card 15, References
ROC Curves - Chart H (Section 3.5)
Sample Size - Section 4.3
Sample Size and Power - see Sample Size
SBAR Technique - Section 6.3

Scatter Plots - Chart G (Section 3.5)
Selection Bias - Section 1.5, Appendix C
Sensitivity & Specificity - Chart H (ROC Curves)
Spin, Glossary of - Section 1.4, Appendix E
Statistical Tests - Section 3.3, Appendix B
Study Designs - Section 1.3, 2.1-2.4
Subgroup Analysis - Chart N
Systematic Reviews - Section 1.3, 2.4
t-Test - Section 3.1, Appendix B
Time Management - Section 6.2
Viva Checklist - Section 6.1
Viva Technique - Section 6

Quick Reference Card — Exam Day!

Chart Recognition (5 seconds)

- **Steps going down?** → Kaplan–Meier
- **Squares with lines?** → Forest Plot
- **Side-by-side bars?** → Bar Chart
- **Slices of circle?** → Pie Chart
- **Box with whiskers?** → Box Plot
- **Dots scattered?** → Scatter Plot
- **Curve to top-left?** → ROC Curve
- **Inverted funnel?** → Funnel Plot
- **Two-by-two grid of counts?** → 2×2 Table (calculate ARR and NNT)
- **Boxes narrowing down the page?** → CONSORT (did analysed match randomised?)
- **Thousands narrowing to dozens?** → PRISMA (how wide was the search?)
- **Curves rising from zero?** → Cumulative Incidence (competing risks)
- **Dots against a 45° line?** → Calibration Plot (is 20% really 20%?)
- **Overall result split by age, sex, stage?** → Subgroup Forest (find the interaction test)
- **Dots inside curved limits, by volume?** → Institutional Funnel (not publication bias)
- **Differences plotted against means, three horizontal lines?** → Bland–Altman (are the limits clinically tolerable?)

Must-Know Formulas

- **ARR** = CER — EER
- **RRR** = ARR / CER
- **NNT** = 1 / ARR
- **RR** = EER / CER
- **OR** = (a×d) / (b×c)
- **Sensitivity** = TP / (TP+FN)
- **Specificity** = TN / (TN+FP)

⚠ Never Say These!

- ~~✗ "Age causes complications"~~
- ~~✗ "p=0.05 so it's important"~~
- ~~✗ "The paper says..."~~
- ~~✗ Guessing rather than admitting uncertainty~~

✓ Say These Instead

- ✓ "Age correlates with..."
- ✓ "Statistically significant but..."
- ✓ "The authors found..."
- ✓ "Based on what I see..."

5-Step Answer Template

1. **Type:** "This is a [chart type]"
2. **Shows:** "Comparing [X] vs [Y]"
3. **Key finding:** "[Main result with numbers]"
4. **Significance:** "p=[value], CI=[range]"
5. **Interpretation:** "Clinically, this means…"

Interpreting Any Statistical Result

P-Values:
$p<0.001$ = a smaller p-value, not a larger or more important effect
$p<0.05$ = statistically significant, which is not the same as clinically important
$p \geq 0.05$ = no conventional evidence against the null at the 5% level — not proof of no effect
Confidence Intervals:
Differences: Crosses 0? → NS
Ratios: Crosses 1? → NS
Narrow = precise
Effect Sizes:
Always give ARR + NNT
Don't quote RRR alone
Context matters!

30-Minute Reading Period Strategy

0-4 min:
Orientation — abstract, design, main result
4-16 min:
Interrogation — PICO, Table 1, main results, CIs
16-24 min:
Construction — 2 strengths, 2 limitations, NNT, clinical application
24-29 min:
Rehearsal — say the opening silently, ready your first two answers, pick your number, decide your closing line
You've got this! Stay calm, stay structured, show them what you know.

References

1. Cunningham D, et al. Perioperative chemotherapy versus surgery alone for resectable gastro-oesophageal cancer. N Engl J Med. 2006;355:11-20. (MAGIC Trial)
2. van Hagen P, et al. Preoperative chemoradiotherapy for oesophageal or junctional cancer. N Engl J Med. 2012;366:2074-2084. (CROSS Trial) — long-term follow-up: Shapiro J, et al. Lancet Oncol. 2015;16:1090-1098.
3. Giuliano AE, et al. Axillary dissection vs no axillary dissection in women with invasive breast cancer and sentinel node metastasis. JAMA. 2011;305:569-575. (ACOSOG Z0011) — 10-year outcomes: Giuliano AE, et al. JAMA. 2017;318:918-926.
4. Giuliano AE, Ballman K, McCall L, et al. Locoregional recurrence after sentinel lymph node dissection with or without axillary dissection in patients with sentinel lymph node metastases: long-term follow-up from the American College of Surgeons Oncology Group (Alliance) ACOSOG Z0011 randomized trial. Ann Surg. 2016;264(3):413-420. (ACOSOG Z0011 — locoregional recurrence)
5. Kapiteijn E, et al. Preoperative radiotherapy combined with total mesorectal excision for resectable rectal cancer. N Engl J Med. 2001;345:638-646. (Dutch TME Trial) — 12-year follow-up: van Gijn W, et al. Lancet Oncol. 2011;12:575-582.
6. Al-Batran SE, et al. Perioperative chemotherapy with fluorouracil plus leucovorin, oxaliplatin, and docetaxel versus fluorouracil or capecitabine plus cisplatin and epirubicin for locally advanced, resectable gastric or gastro-oesophageal junction adenocarcinoma (FLOT4): a randomised, phase 2/3 trial. Lancet. 2019;393:1948-1957.
7. Hoeppner J, et al. Perioperative chemotherapy (FLOT) versus preoperative chemoradiotherapy (CROSS) in resectable oesophageal adenocarcinoma (ESOPEC): a randomised, controlled trial. N Engl J Med. 2025;392:323-335. DOI: 10.1056/NEJMoa2409408.
8. Reynolds JV, et al. Trimodality therapy versus perioperative chemotherapy in the management of locally advanced adenocarcinoma of the oesophagus and oesophagogastric junction (Neo-AEGIS): an open-label, randomised, phase 3 trial. Lancet Gastroenterol Hepatol. 2023;8(11):1015-1027. (Neo-AEGIS Trial)
9. Kato K, et al. Doublet chemotherapy, triplet chemotherapy, or doublet chemotherapy combined with radiotherapy as neoadjuvant treatment for locally advanced oesophageal cancer (JCOG1109 NExT): a randomised, controlled, open-label, phase 3 trial. Lancet. 2024;404(10447):55-66. DOI: 10.1016/S0140-6736(24)00745-1. (JCOG1109 / NExT Trial)
10. Neoptolemos JP, et al. Comparison of adjuvant gemcitabine and capecitabine with gemcitabine monotherapy in patients with resected

pancreatic cancer (ESPAC-4): a multicentre, open-label, randomised, phase 3 trial. Lancet. 2017;389:1011-1024.
11. Conroy T, et al. FOLFIRINOX or gemcitabine as adjuvant therapy for pancreatic cancer (PRODIGE-24/CCTG PA6). N Engl J Med. 2018;379:2395-2406.
12. Bonjer HJ, et al. A randomized trial of laparoscopic versus open surgery for rectal cancer (COLOR II). N Engl J Med. 2015;372:1324-1332.
13. Guillou PJ, et al. Short-term endpoints of conventional versus laparoscopic-assisted surgery in patients with colorectal cancer (MRC CLASICC trial): multicentre, randomised controlled trial. Lancet. 2005;365:1718-1726.
14. Jayne DG, Thorpe HC, Copeland J, Quirke P, Brown JM, Guillou PJ. Five-year follow-up of the Medical Research Council CLASICC trial of laparoscopically assisted versus open surgery for colorectal cancer. Br J Surg. 2010;97(11):1638-1645. (CLASICC long-term outcomes)
15. Mansel RE, et al. Randomized multicenter trial of sentinel node biopsy versus standard axillary treatment in operable breast cancer: the ALMANAC Trial. J Natl Cancer Inst. 2006;98:599-609.
16. Sparano JA, et al. Adjuvant chemotherapy guided by a 21-gene expression assay in breast cancer (TAILORx). N Engl J Med. 2018;379:111-121.
17. Greenhalgh T. How to read a paper: The basics of evidence-based medicine. 6th ed. Wiley-Blackwell; 2019.
18. Sackett DL, et al. Evidence-based medicine: How to practice and teach EBM. 2nd ed. Churchill Livingstone; 2000.
19. Centre for Evidence-Based Medicine. Oxford Centre for Evidence-Based Medicine: Levels of Evidence (2009). Available at: https://www.cebm.ox.ac.uk (Note: GRADE — Grading of Recommendations, Assessment, Development and Evaluations — is an alternative certainty-of-evidence framework increasingly referenced in clinical guidelines; some FRCS examiners may prefer this framework to traditional Oxford levels.)
20. Moher D, et al. CONSORT 2010 explanation and elaboration: updated guidelines for reporting parallel group randomised trials. BMJ. 2010;340:c869.
21. Hopewell S, et al. CONSORT 2025 explanation and elaboration: updated guideline for reporting randomised trials. BMJ. 2025;389:e081124.
22. Hopewell S, et al. CONSORT 2025 statement: updated guideline for reporting randomised trials. BMJ. 2025;389:e081123.
23. Schulz KF, Grimes DA. Blinding in randomised trials: hiding who got what. Lancet. 2002;359:696-700.
24. Altman DG, Bland JM. How to obtain the P value from a confidence interval. BMJ. 2011;343:d2304.

25. Cook JA, et al. DELTA2 guidance on choosing the target difference and undertaking and reporting the sample size calculation for a randomised controlled trial. BMJ. 2018;363:k3750.
26. Higgins JPT, Thomas J, Chandler J, Cumpston M, Li T, Page MJ, Welch VA (editors). Cochrane Handbook for Systematic Reviews of Interventions Version 6.5. Cochrane, 2024.
27. Jüni P, et al. Systematic reviews in health care: Assessing the quality of controlled clinical trials. BMJ. 2001;323:42-6.
28. Schulz KF, et al. Empirical evidence of bias: dimensions of methodological quality associated with estimates of treatment effects in controlled trials. JAMA. 1995;273:408-412.
29. Montori VM, et al. Randomised controlled trials. In: Guyatt G, et al, editors. Users' Guides to the Medical Literature. 3rd ed. McGraw-Hill; 2015.
30. Grimes DA, Schulz KF. Cohort studies: marching towards outcomes. Lancet. 2002;359:341-5.
31. Schulz KF, Grimes DA. Case-control studies: research in reverse. Lancet. 2002;359:431-4.
32. Sedgwick P. Pitfalls of statistical hypothesis testing: multiple testing. BMJ. 2014;349:g5310.
33. Sterne JAC, et al. RoB 2: a revised tool for assessing risk of bias in randomised trials. BMJ. 2019;366:l4898.
34. Guyatt GH, et al. GRADE: an emerging consensus on rating quality of evidence and strength of recommendations. BMJ. 2008;336:924-6.
35. Akobeng AK. Understanding diagnostic tests 2: likelihood ratios, pre- and post-test probabilities and their use in clinical practice. Acta Paediatr. 2007;96:487-491.
36. Page MJ, et al. The PRISMA 2020 statement: an updated guideline for reporting systematic reviews. BMJ. 2021;372:n71.
37. Egger M, Davey Smith G, Schneider M, Minder C. Bias in meta-analysis detected by a simple, graphical test. BMJ. 1997;315:629-634.
38. Duval S, Tweedie R. Trim and fill: a simple funnel-plot-based method of testing and adjusting for publication bias in meta-analysis. Biometrics. 2000;56:455-463.
39. Bland JM, Altman DG. Statistical methods for assessing agreement between two methods of clinical measurement. Lancet. 1986;1:307-310.
40. Joint Committee on Intercollegiate Examinations (JCIE). Regulations relating to the Intercollegiate Specialty Examination in General Surgery. Policy SR5 v8.0, last reviewed Aug 2025. Available at: https://www.jcie.org.uk
41. Joint Committee on Intercollegiate Examinations (JCIE). Section 2 Marking Descriptors. Available at: https://www.jcie.org.uk
42. Joint Committee on Intercollegiate Examinations (JCIE). Regulations relating to the Intercollegiate Specialty Examination in Vascular Surgery.

Policy SR13 v8.0, last reviewed Aug 2025. Available at: https://www.jcie.org.uk

About the Author

J. R. Morgan is the pen name of a practising surgeon with more than twenty years of experience. Drawing on that experience, this handbook distils what the FRCS academic viva actually rewards — clear appraisal, calm judgement, and the right words under pressure — into a method you can rehearse.
Part of the AMaC series: think like an examiner, speak like a doctor, perform with confidence.

About This Book

The FRCS Part 2 academic viva doesn't reward the trainee who memorised the most — it rewards the one who can pick up an unfamiliar paper, find the flaw that matters, and say so with the confidence of a consultant. This handbook teaches exactly that. Inside: the frameworks examiners look for, five-second recognition drills for every chart type you'll be handed, worked critiques of the landmark trials, a Glossary of Spin that decodes what a paper is really saying, and a Test Yourself set to rehearse against. Think like an examiner, speak like a doctor, perform with confidence.

Good Luck!

You've worked hard to get here.
Trust your preparation.
Stay calm, stay structured, and show them what you know.
Remember AMaC's philosophy:
"Making the Difficult Easy"
J.R. Morgan · AMaC Publishing
FRCS Part 2 Paper Critique Handbook
2026 Edition